Mindful Places to Stay

Sublime Destinations for Yoga and Meditation

gestalten

CONTENTS

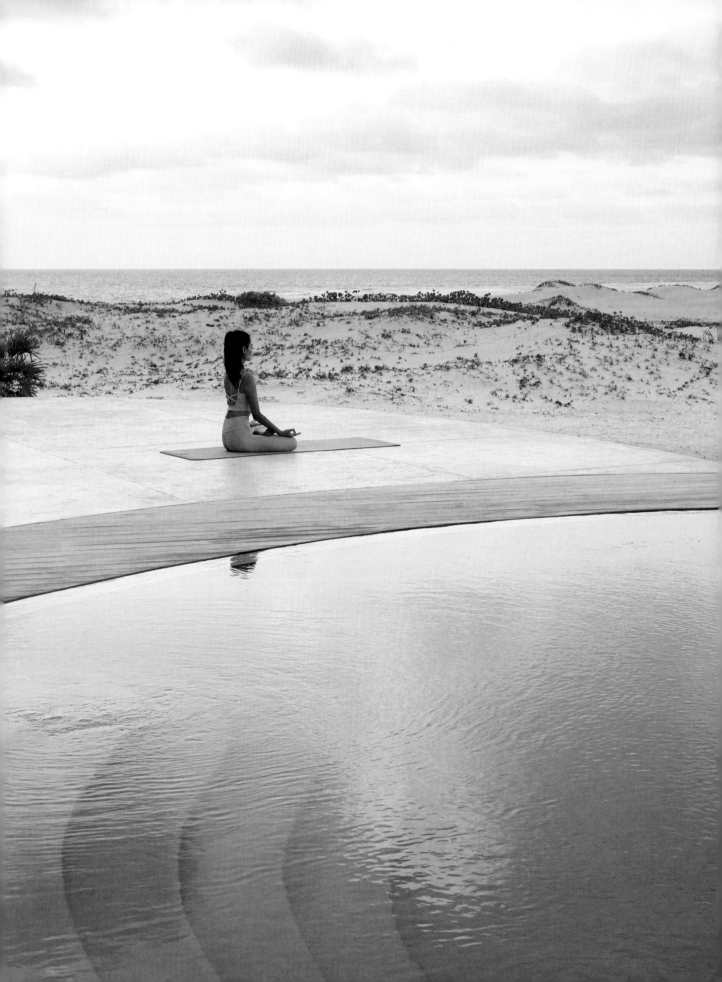

TRANQUIL SPACES IN WHICH TO NURTURE YOUR MENTAL, EMOTIONAL, AND SPIRITUAL WELL-BEING

The world's most idyllic retreats in remote places—spaces for reconnecting with nature and, ultimately, yourself

When we dream about the perfect vacation destination, many of us are thinking beyond simply taking time off work. We are looking for a retreat that offers a deeper, longer-lasting impact, be it spiritual, physical, or creative. We seek to nourish our minds and bodies with soulful meditation and healthful foods. And we want to return home well rested and rejuvenated—changed. All across the globe are vacation places dedicated solely to our physical and mental health—resorts and retreats in peaceful, natural surroundings that encourage us to slow down, to take a breath, and to indulge in a little personal introspection. Their bucolic settings allow us to reconnect with nature and to spend quality time with like-minded people, participating in activities known for their positive effects on our well-being. That could be taking a communal yoga class, relaxing in a hydro-therapy tank, learning an artisanal craft, or harvesting locally grown ingredients for a wholesome meal.

What counts as an ideal retreat varies widely from one person to the next. For some, it might be a few days at a wholesome yoga school; for others, a program of therapeutic massages might be the answer. But what they all have in common, is the opportunity to engage in an transformative experience that promotes deep self-reflection—a period without distraction that allows us to de-stress, reenergize, and return home feeling totally at one with ourselves.

Key to all the retreats that feature in this book is the beauty of their location. Though found in every corner of the world, from the cacti-strewn Baja California desert in Mexico to the foothills of the Franschhoek mountains in South Africa to the Balinese

OPPOSITE At the Kisawa Sanctuary, guests can swim or simply spend a tranquil moment next to the idyllic organically shaped pool.

5

tropical rain forest, these 29 resorts and boutique hotels occupy land in the most idyllic of natural surroundings. Some span vast areas of unspoiled land with private beaches; others are tucked away among acres of woodland, some perch on the terraces of lush mountain valleys, and others sit at the heart of the most stunning landscaped gardens. Each and every one of them promises peace and tranquility from dawn till dusk and a stillness that guests would find hard to achieve at home. Within hours of arrival, they feel at one with their surroundings, keenly aware of nature's rhythm and in tune with the local wildlife. There are paths and trails to explore and plenty of private spaces in which to sit in quiet contemplation.

The architecture, too, is carefully considered and designed in such a way that it blends in with its environment. Whether guests are looking for a lakeside cabin, a stone cottage in the country, or a beachfront yurt, every imaginable scenario is possible. A retreat hub might be a repurposed farm, monastery, or fortress steeped in local history and carefully restored to suit its new role while retaining key features from its past life. Where resorts are more contemporary, accommodation often blends in with its surroundings, supporting the immersive quality of the guests' experience. At the Japanese retreat KAI Yufuin Hoshino (p. 64), rooms are situated in a traditional Japanese inn, or *ryokan*, surrounded by rice terraces, for example, while at the Suenyo

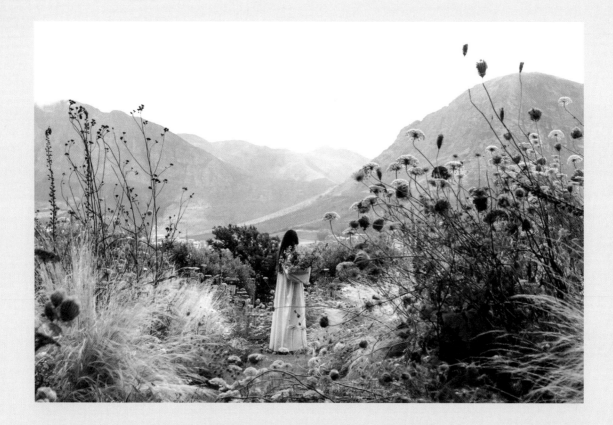

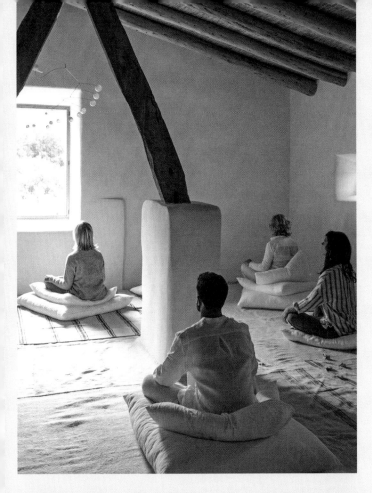

Eco Retreat, in Bali (p. 86), elegant, sculptural bamboo pavilions appear almost suspended from the trees.

Ranging from single- and double-occupancy rooms to entire suites and standalone villas, accommodation is always comfortable, sometimes even luxurious, but is usually sparsely decorated so as not to distract guests. Furnished simply and dressed using natural textiles in neutral tones, they offer spaces of optimum calm. Many have ensuite bathrooms stocked with top-quality organic bathing products, private decks with hot tubs, and terraces or balconies with stunning views. They all have isolated spaces for relaxation and contemplation. As such, they encourage deep restorative sleep by night, while inspiring contemplation and creativity by day. Common to each retreat's public spaces are beautiful gardens, generous lounges with wood-burning stoves, indoor and outdoor swimming pools, sun terraces, and decks with fire pits for convivial evening gatherings and gazing at the stars.

Almost all of the resorts have their own restaurants, many of them following the farm-to-table tradition of menus based on local, seasonal produce. In a bid to offer holistic experiences, many venues promote health-giving vegan and vegetarian menus that support a particular wellness program.

When it comes to the transformative experience, the retreats in this book fall broadly into two categories: those with a focus on yoga, breathing exercises, and meditation, and those with spas for health treatments ranging from massages and body wraps to sound baths and saunas. Among the yoga

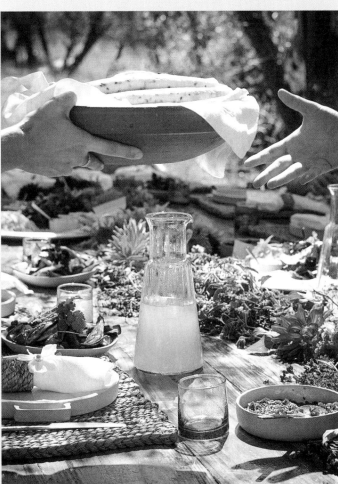

OPPOSITE AND LEFT From morning yoga to the daily harvest, activities focused on movement, creativity, and play interweave through the day at Sterrekopje Farm. TOP A meditation class at Es Racó d'Artà on the Spanish island of Mallorca.

retreats, Silver Island Yoga in Greece (p. 24) offers classes in a yoga *shala* overlooking the Aegean Sea. Under the direction of a dynamic group of instructors guests can choose from a wide range of yoga styles at every level from beginner to advanced. At Vale de Moses in central Portugal (p. 70), each day starts with a group yoga session and in the afternoons guests attend workshops on different aspects of the yogic way of life. If you are booked in to stay at Raga Svara (p. 58) in India, you can preselect your retreat options, all of which are designed to target specific areas such as stress and weight management or women's health. Each program blends the spiritual with the physical and includes a daily schedule of Ayurvedic therapies, yoga classes, breathing techniques, and meditation sessions, supported by a personalized dietary regime.

At the spa-based resorts, many of the most popular therapies have origins in traditional Ayurvedic and Chinese practices, but other practices are also offered alongside them. At the lakeside retreat Villa Sumaya (p. 230) in the Guatemalan highlands, for example, treatments include Reiki, reflexology, and acupuncture alongside Swedish neuro-lumbar massage, deep tissue massage, and facial treatments. Building on the Latvian sauna tradition, the Latvian Ziedlejas nature spa (p. 150) offers deeply relaxing, personal bathing sessions in one of the retreat's three unique saunas. Each guest is treated to a three-to-four-hour session surrounded by fragrant plants, with a personal masseur who applies a range of therapies for the body using warm air and besoms.

To complement their program—whether one primarily of yoga/meditation or physical therapy/massage—most retreats offer additional activities that are equally uplifting for mind, body, and soul. These can include anything from cookering and pottery classes to jewelry-making courses, hiking in the surrounding countryside, forest bathing, and wild swimming. There are also options for anyone seeking professional help on a more physical level. Es Racó d'Artà in Mallorca, Spain (p. 18), is a certified wellness center offering deep-healing *watsu* and *wata* therapies—Zen shiatsu-inspired bodywork that takes place while you are floating in warm water.

It is not unusual for a resort to facilitate some sort of learning during a stay. Many have well-stocked libraries full of books on well-being so that guests can gain a deeper insight to relaxation and meditation practices and discover new ways of healing naturally. Others provide hands-on farming tutorials or cooking classes to encourage guests to take new practices home with them and use them to make positive changes in their diet and lifestyle. It is through such measures that the transformative experience comes full circle, providing guests with lasting techniques for improving their well-being on a daily basis. Each story in this book is accompanied with stunning photographs of the retreats, the activities they have to offer, and unspoiled views across valleys, lush forests, and out to sea. As you read from one to the next, you can almost feel the warm sun on your face and sense the calm that inhabits your body through gentle meditation. Take your time and, page after page, the act of reading might even provide a transformative, immersive experience of its own.   ✳

OPPOSITE Inviting paths wind through the lush tropical jungle at the COMO Shambhala Estate holistic wellness sanctuary, Bali.

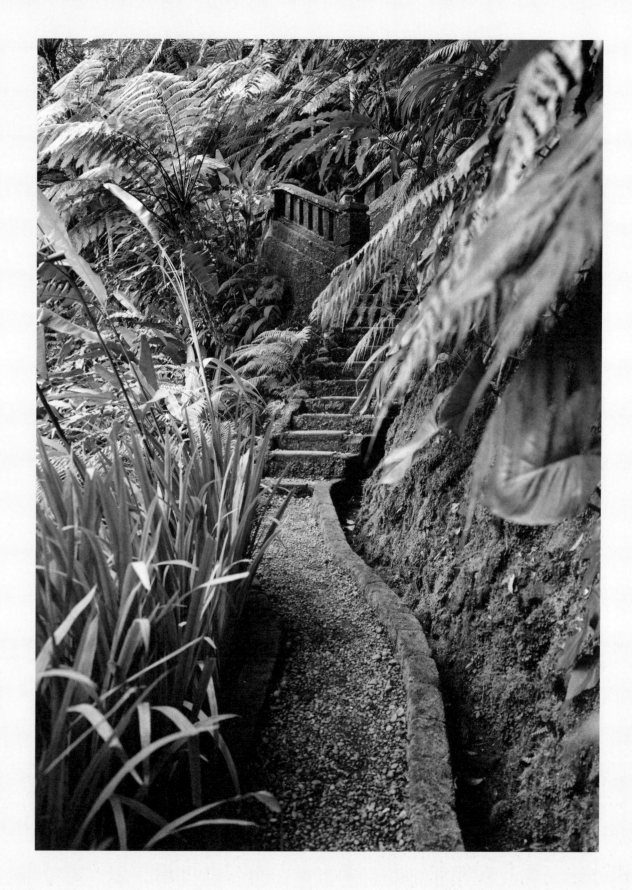

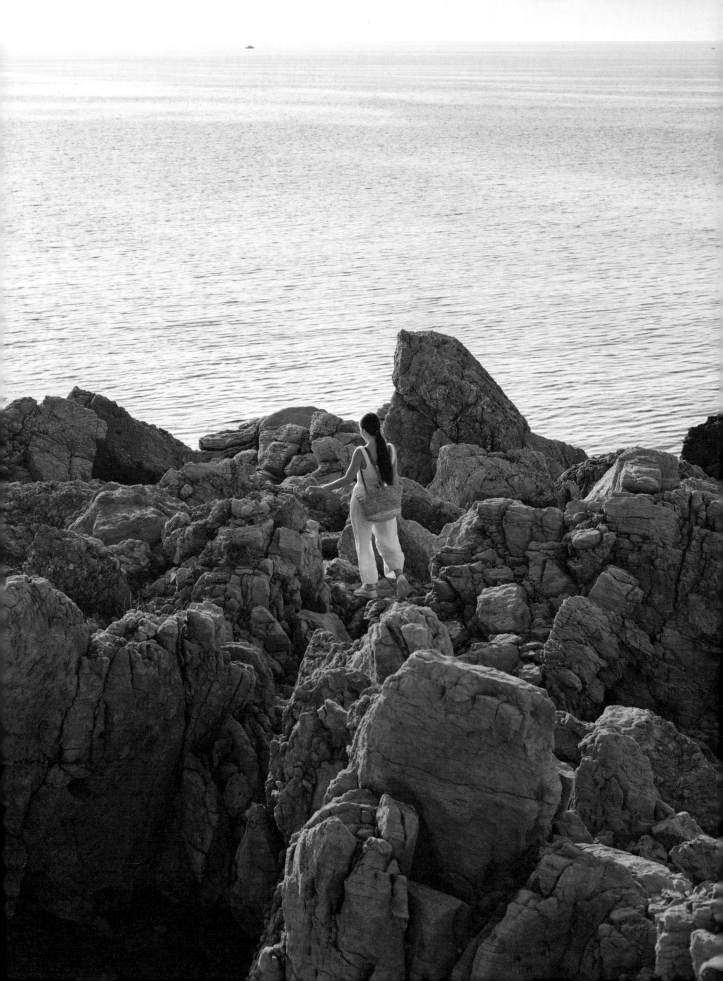

A GATHERING OF WOMEN FOR
WHOM THE INNER JOURNEY
IS AS IMPORTANT AS THE OUTER

she she Retreats
Deià, Mallorca, Spain

A Mallorcan HILLTOP MONASTERY is the setting for a women-only late-summer retreat. With no more than 11 guests at a time, the focus is on SHARED EXPERIENCE and going with the flow.

The retreats promise to deliver "mindful, community-centered sojourns." Guests are invited to come together in locations of rugged beauty across Europe, arriving "only with an open mind." For four nights and five days, women take part in activities including movement, silent practice, workshops, excursions, and shared meals. With an emphasis on adventure and slowness, there is no fixed agenda. Events are navigated through intuition, serendipity, and connection.

This 13th-century Mallorcan monastery is one of several retreat locations, which also include a guest house on the Italian island of Pantelleria and a farmhouse in the foothills of the German Alps. The monastery is perched above the village of Deià, which lies in the Tramuntana mountain range running parallel to the island's northwest coast. With breathtaking views of the Mediterranean and surrounded by ancient olive groves, the area has been an inspiration to artists, writers, and musicians for centuries. Brimming with the charm of a rural home, the property itself has welcoming communal spaces that include a cozy living room and an outdoor terrace with an infinity pool. There are also numerous nooks and crannies in which guests can enjoy the sweet scent of citrus trees or catch the sun dipping below the horizon come dusk. The resort offers a diverse and balanced program with different practices for body and mind. The day typically starts with a period of silence, during which there is no conversation, no screen time, and no reading. A series of dynamic movement sessions take place during the day, while in the evening there is a mixture of meditation, restorative

OPPOSITE Many of the activities at she she Retreats are shared experiences with like-minded women. There is also plenty of time for self-reflection inspired by the island's rugged beauty.

movement, and calming bedtime rituals. Mealtimes are rooted in the philosophy that what we eat and how we eat is a reflection of the relationship we form with ourselves. An all-female team focuses on thoughtful eating experiences, merging cooking techniques with an aesthetic of beautiful simplicity and wholesomeness. The dynamic vegetarian menu combines local and seasonal ingredients, and each serving comes from careful consideration of the whole journey of the food, from the root to the table. Guests are mostly women traveling alone, with a wide range of ages and from diverse backgrounds. They share bedrooms and daily activities with one another in an intimate environment without judgment or preconceptions and in which all are equal. Inevitably, they form a sense of sisterhood that is inspiring, transformative, and empowering.　＊

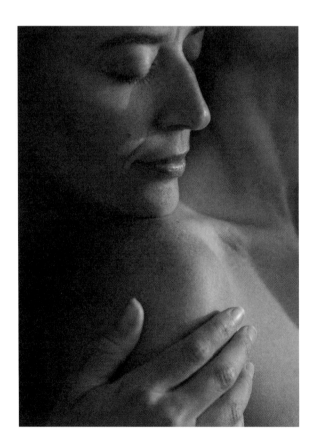
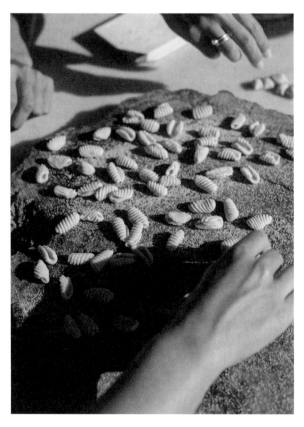

ABOVE In the belief that well-being extends far beyond purely physical activity, each stay includes a creative workshop, a cooking workshop, and a self-care workshop. OPPOSITE The simple, honest architecture of the Mallorcan retreat helps to create a sense of calm.

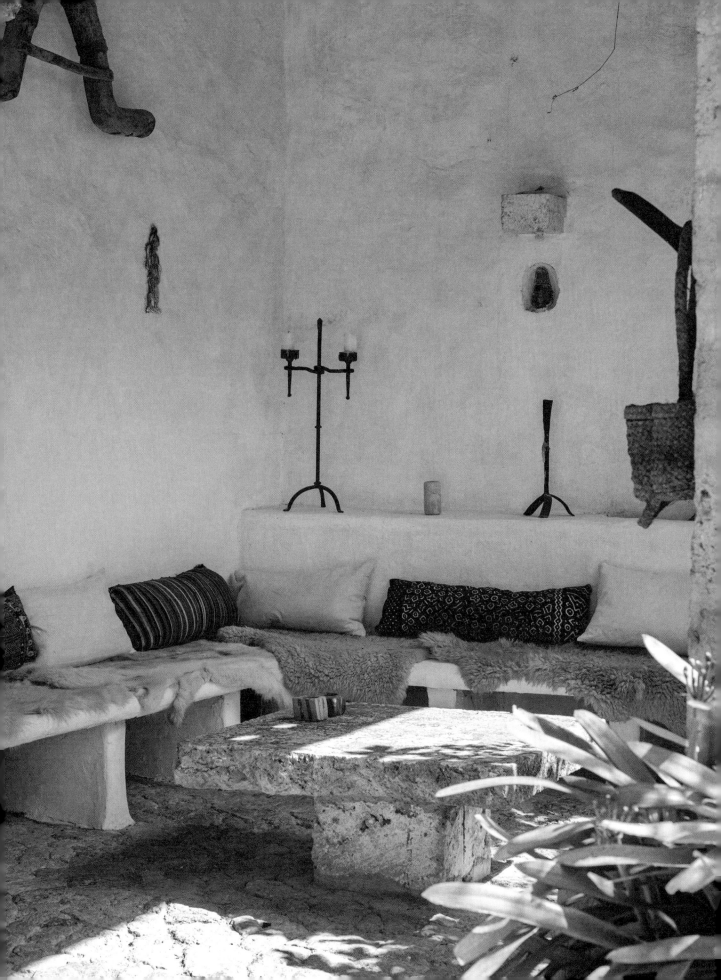

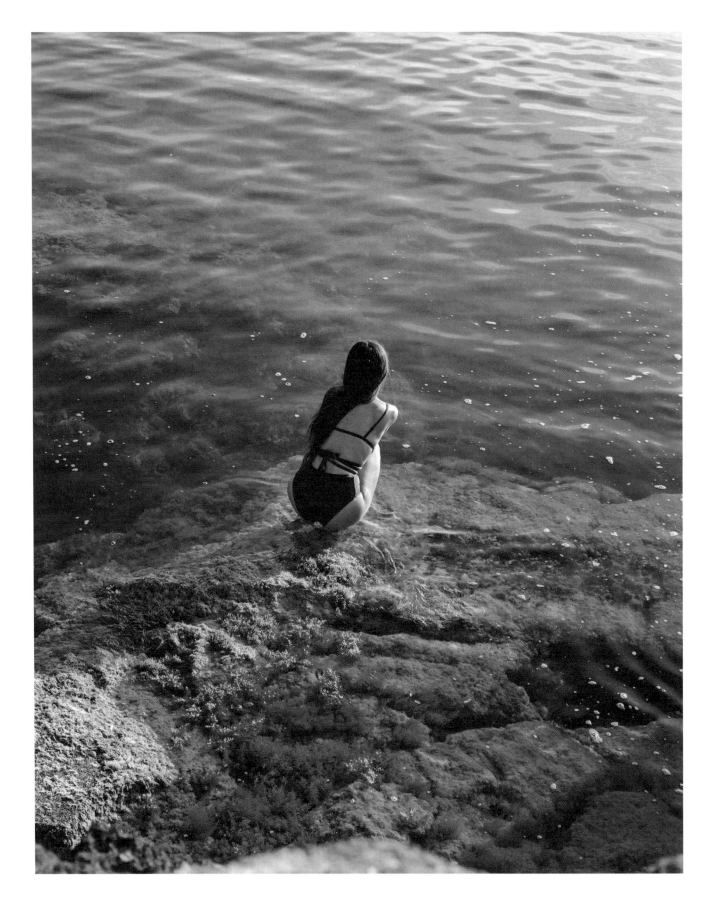

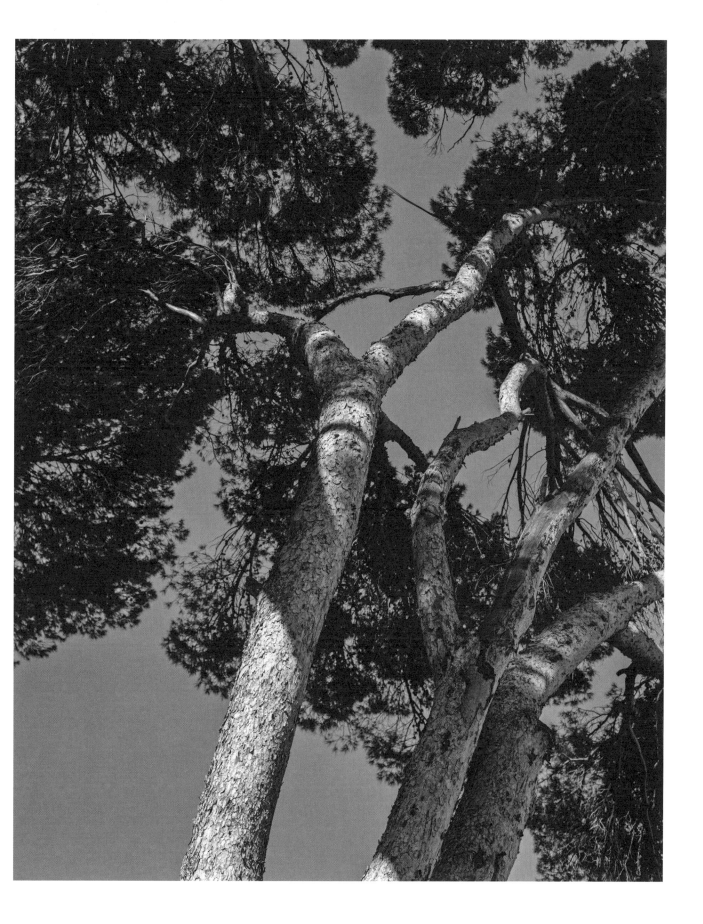

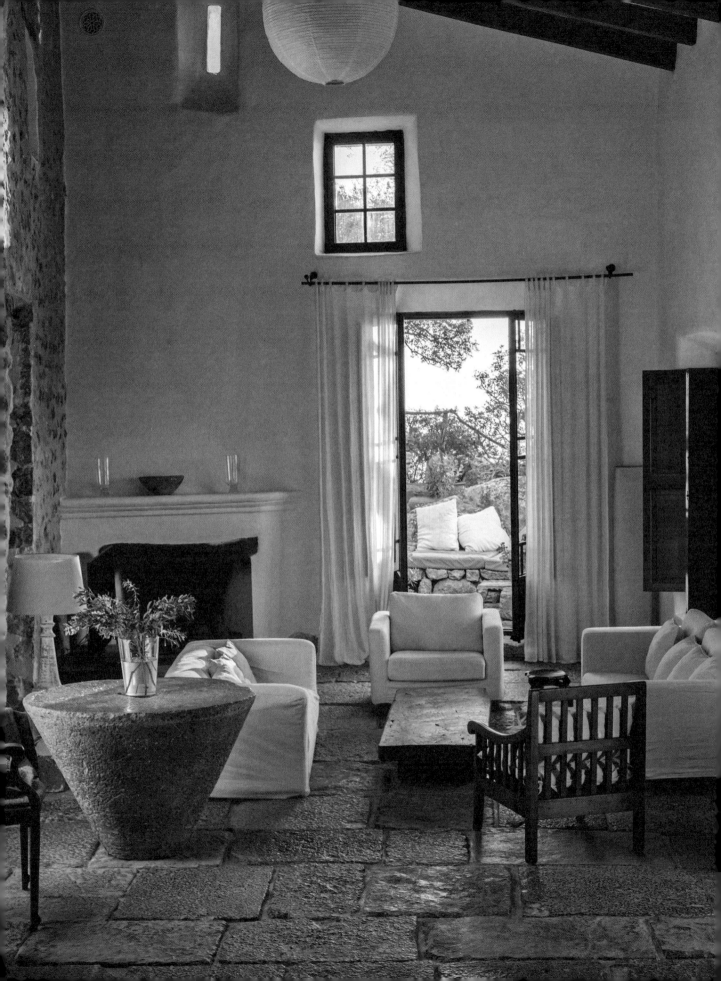

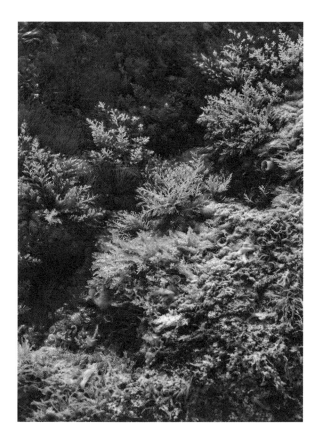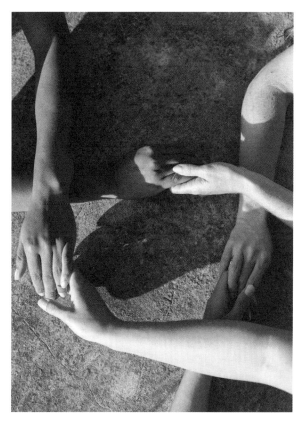

OPPOSITE Much of the original aesthetic of the former monastery in the Tramuntana mountain range has been retained—
the beamed ceilings, whitewashed walls, stone floors, and furnishings are made from natural materials in neutral colors.

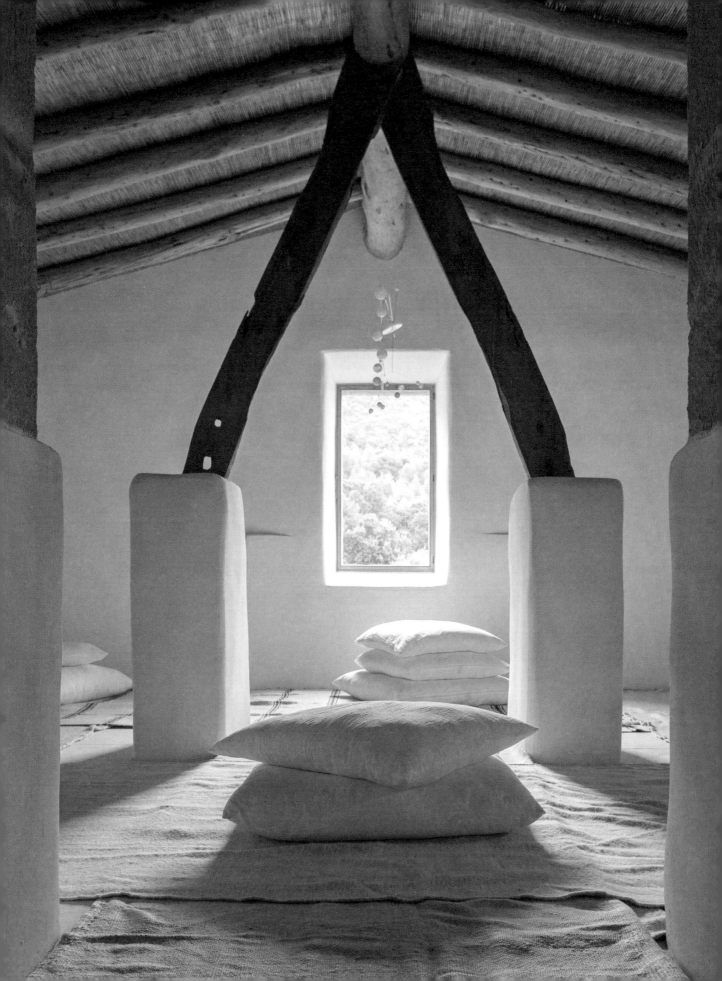

A DESTINATION FOR TRANSFORMATION THAT PROMISES TO REJUVENATE MIND, BODY, AND SPIRIT

Es Racó d'Artà

Artà, Mallorca, Spain

Focusing on HOLISTIC PRACTICES *and* TOTAL IMMERSION *in quiet, natural surroundings, this Mallorcan wellness center offers signature retreats dedicated to the relationship between* NATURE AND SOCIETY.

Es Racó d'Artà is nestled in a serene valley on the Llevant peninsula in northeast Mallorca, a spot that is stunning all year round. It provides a tranquil refuge in which guests are encouraged to "experience, discover, feel, and express through art, movement, silence, meditation, reflection, and rich conversation," and are invited to rest their minds, open their hearts, and nurture their bodies.

Surrounded by mountains and within walking distance of the pretty village of Artà and the turquoise Mediterranean Sea, Es Racó d'Artà finca occupies 540 acres (220 hectares) of land that include forests of oak, wild olive, carob, pine, and cypress as well as a 35-acre (14-hectare) ecological vineyard, olive groves, fruit orchards, an organic vegetable garden, and aromatic herbal garden. Choice of accommodation varies considerably across the resort and includes a house and a range of double rooms, suites, and woodland cottages—many with private terraces and pools. The maximum capacity is 68 guests.

Proudly proclaiming to be "a destination for transformation," Es Racó d'Artà is a certified wellness center offering a wide range of deep-healing therapies that include *watsu* and *wata* treatments—Zen shiatsu-inspired bodywork that takes place while you're floating in warm water—as well as many forms of massage, yoga, and meditation. The treatments are designed to awaken the senses, transporting guests to a realm of tranquility and luxury. Working in a sanctuary powered by geothermal technology, the expert therapists use locally sourced, natural cosmetic products, demonstrating that luxury and

OPPOSITE The retreat stands on an estate that was once a working farm. This simple outhouse was transformed into a serene and lofty space for meaningful meditation.

responsible environmental stewardship can coexist seamlessly.

The same philosophy is at the heart of the center's approach to gastronomy, which focuses on seasonal, locally grown organic produce. This, plus an emphasis on Mediterranean cuisine, enables guests to truly appreciate their connection with the surroundings—a key feature of an experience here, according to the owners, Antoni Esteva and Jaume Danús. They want their guests to be inspired by genuine Mallorcan life.

In order to benefit most from the spa, the restaurant, and activities on offer, and to achieve a state of deep relaxation, the owners recommend a three-day stay. Visiting Es Racó d'Artà is not about "checking out" feeling refreshed and relaxed, they say. It is about "checking in" with oneself and with others. It is about "leaning in, deepening, returning to the body, to our senses, to our humanness, fully embodying life here on Earth." ✳

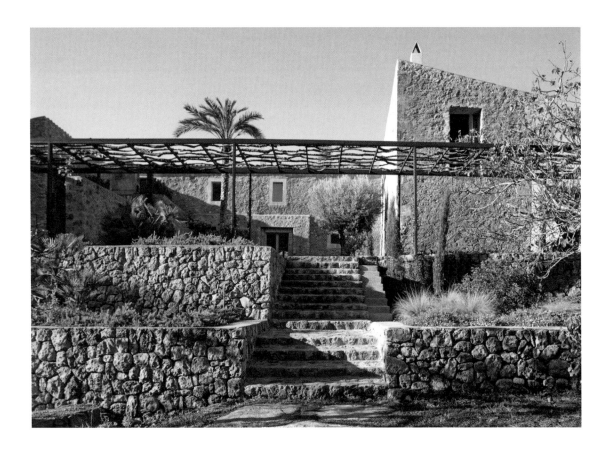

ABOVE AND OPPOSITE The estate finca and other buildings on the site date back to the 13th century. The owners have done much to preserve not just the original footprint of the buildings, but also their original fabric to minimize the impact of their retreat on the natural surroundings.

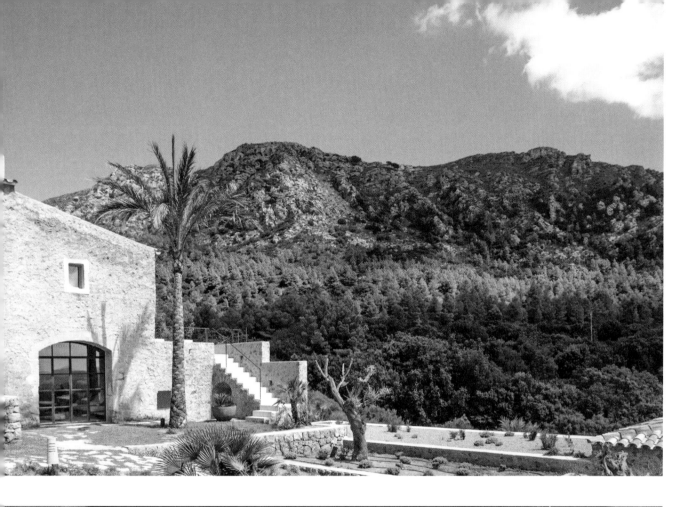

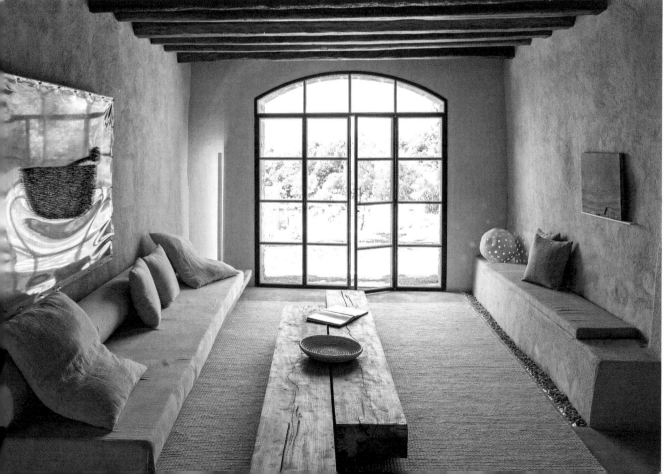

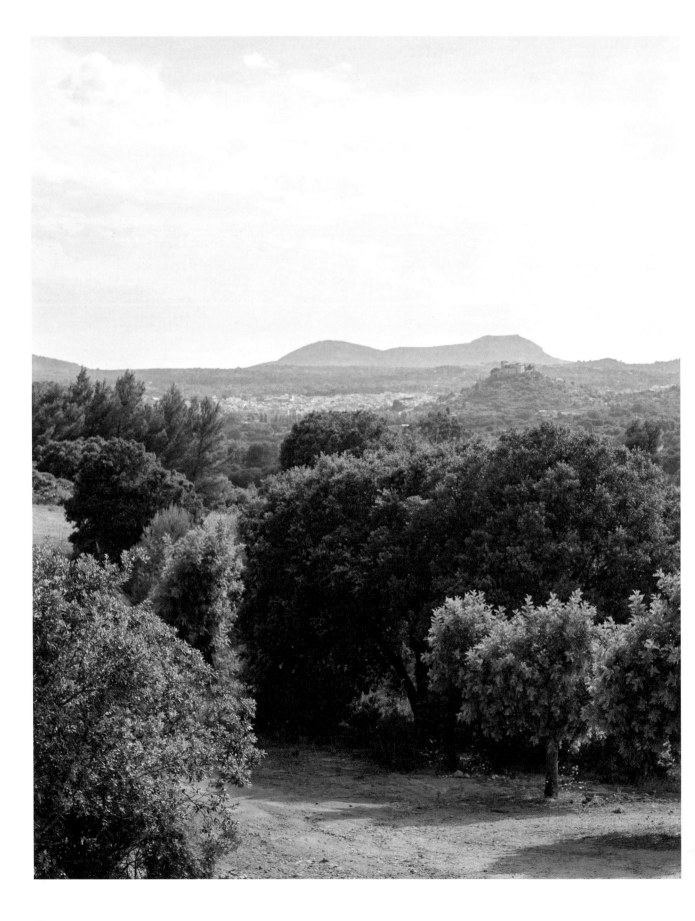

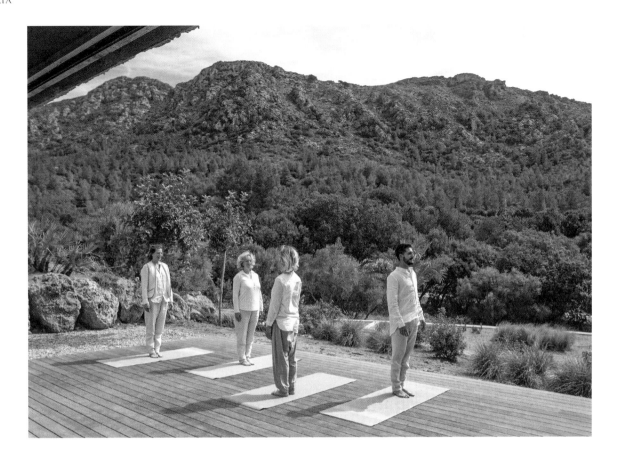

ABOVE Guests take part in a yoga nidra class on the outdoor terrace. Throughout the year, Es Racó d'Artà hosts
retreats with guest practitioners who make maximum use of the site's facilities. These frequently have a singular focus,
such as "recharge and connect" and "women's health."

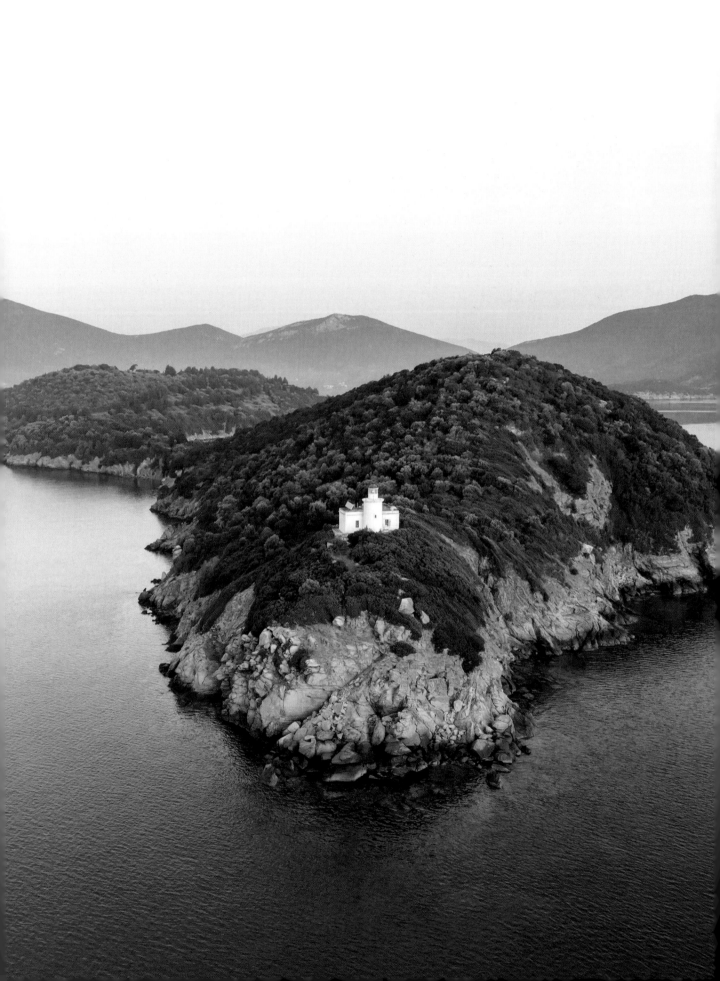

Silver Island Yoga
Silver Island, Greece

RECHARGE YOUR BATTERIES WITH A REJUVENATING EXPERIENCE ON A PRIVATE ISLAND

If you are in search of an escape from the hustle and bustle of modern life, this Silver Island retreat focuses on yoga as a means to inspire INNER PEACE, *abundance, serenity, and* MINDFUL LIVING.

Silver Island lies surrounded by the crystal blue Aegean Sea just northeast of Athens, Greece. With 60 acres (24 hectares) of gently rolling hills, hidden coves, ancient olive groves, and glorious views in all directions, it is a truly magical place in which to merge nature and self. Established by the Christie family in 2013, the center offers weeklong retreats from Sunday through Saturday from mid-April to mid-October.

With just six rooms, housed in a 19th-century home and a 20th-century villa, the center receives a maximum of 12 guests at a time. Bedrooms are well-equipped with complimentary water bottles, slippers, natural toiletries, towels, and beach sarongs. Several rooms have private bathrooms and terraces; all of them have spectacular sea views. Communal spaces include an dining room with a working fireplace, an inviting living room, and an outside eating area and fire pit. A path from the villa leads to a yoga *shala*, a peaceful place for practicing, with magnificent views across the Aegean Sea.

The center prides itself on the standard of its yoga instructors. Handpicked from all around the world, they have many years of experience between them and offer yoga styles to suit everyone's needs, from beginner to advanced. Some of them offer additional therapeutic practices. There is an emphasis on the client choosing how they spend their time at the retreat, joining classes as and when they wish.

Typically, a group yoga class takes place at the open-air *shala* before breakfast is served, after which guests are free to have some beach time, go for a swim, or explore one of the island's many walking paths. Afternoons

OPPOSITE Silver Island, in the Aegean Sea. The resort hosts organize a water taxi to transport guests to and from the private island and the port of Oreoi on the Greek mainland.

are generally set aside for total relaxation, perhaps with a one-to-one yoga session or therapeutic treatment. Then, as the sun begins to set, the yoga day ends with a meditative group class.

All activities are included in the retreat fee, as are delicious, nutritious vegetarian meals based on the healthy Mediterranean diet and made using seasonal, organic, locally sourced ingredients. Guests come together around two big dining tables, either indoors or outside on the terrace to share breakfast, lunch, and dinner family-style. Throughout the day, water, coffee, and tea are always available and guests can help themselves to fresh fruit and healthy snacks. At the beginning and end of the retreat, the center organizes car transfers to and from the private island.   *

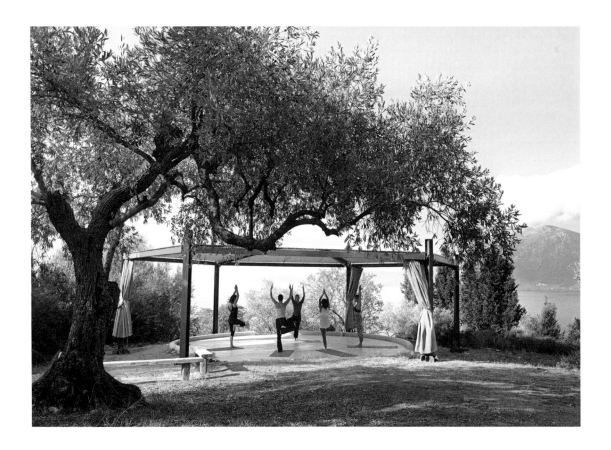

ABOVE AND OPPOSITE Every day at Silver Island Yoga begins and ends in the outdoor yoga *shala*, a shaded platform set beneath an ancient olive tree overlooking the sea. A more active session in the morning and a meditative class come evening allow guests to tune in to the rhythms of the day.

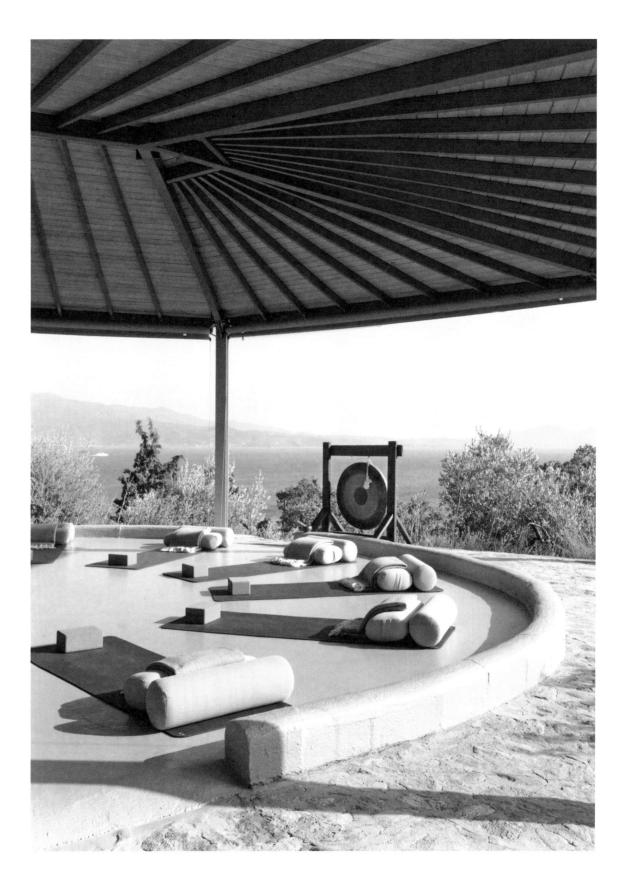

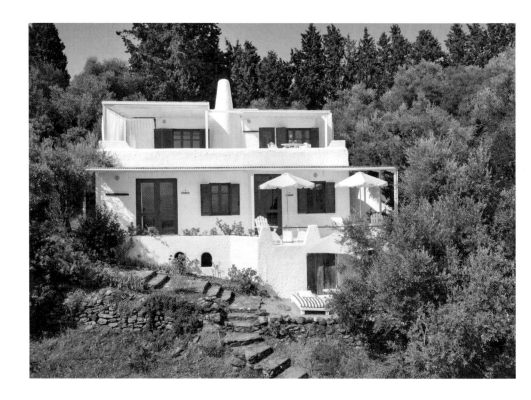

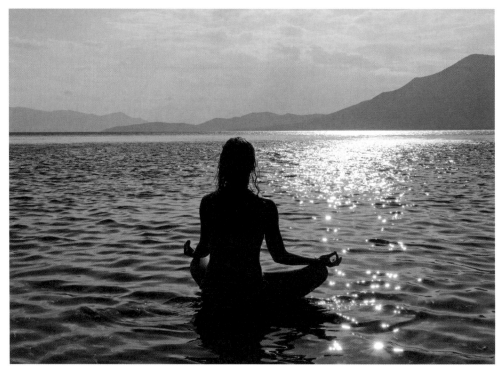

ABOVE AND OPPOSITE Accommodation in the resort's 20th-century villa takes its cue from the traditional Greek village style, with whitewashed walls and floors and blue paintwork. A path leading from the villa takes guests to the yoga *shala* in one direction and to the beach in the other.

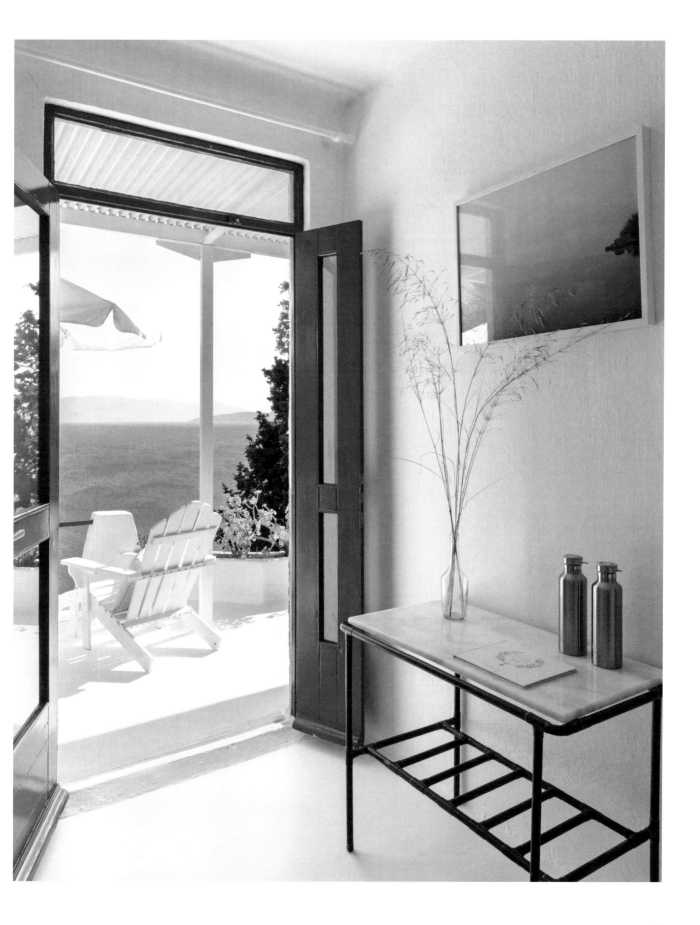

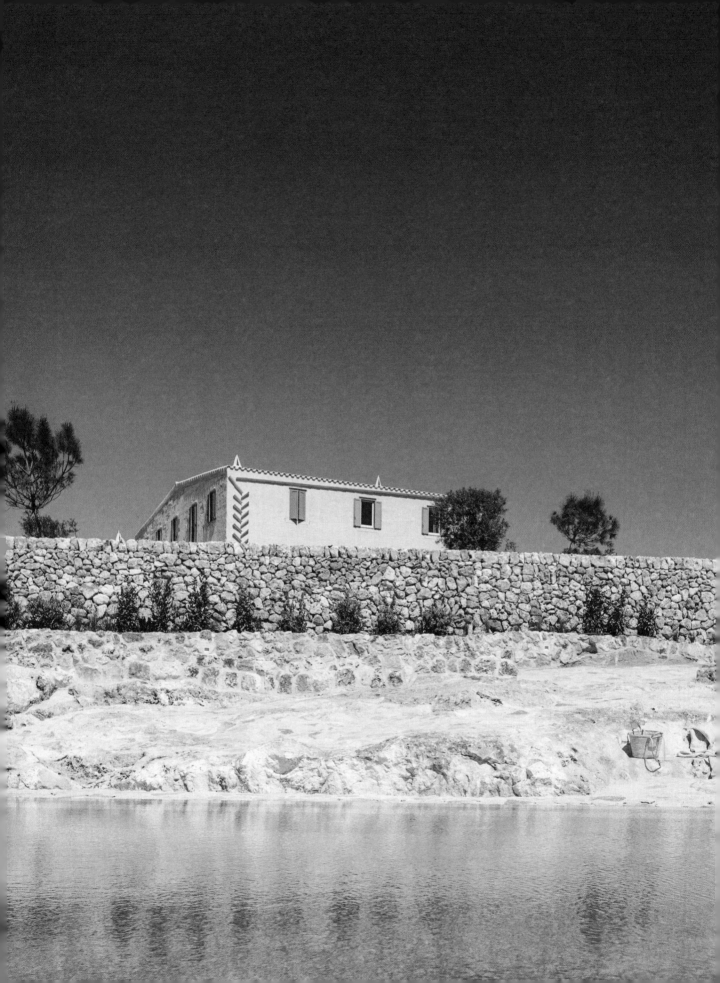

Son Blanc Farmhouse
Menorca, Spain

A UTOPIAN RETREAT FOUNDED ON THE PRINCIPLES OF APPROACHABLE SUSTAINABILITY

Son Blanc Farmhouse invites guests to communicate with NATURE, to reconnect with THEIR OWN ESSENCE, to share moments with GOOD COMPANY, and experience a range of activities intended to UNITE.

Guests staying at Son Blanc on the Spanish island of Menorca quickly find themselves at the heart of a thriving agricultural ecosystem. Practicing self-sufficiency and responsible farming based on crop diversity, resilience, natural productivity, and sustainability, the owners use regenerative agricultural practices to foster communion between nature, their team, and their guests. They have planted thousands of trees and plants on the land and base their cuisine on what it has to offer. Set over an expansive natural reserve, the 320-acre (130-hectare) working farmstead lies in a preserved and wild corner of the island, creating a rare feeling of near total independence among those who stay here. The owners of the retreat have restored and converted a traditional Menorcan farmhouse to accommodate up to 28 guests. Maintaining the charm of the vernacular architecture, they have used local, natural, and sustainable materials throughout to ensure ultra-efficient energy use and natural temperature control. Furnishings are rustic and artisanal and, whether taking clay, stone, or reclaimed wood as inspiration, each of the retreat's 14 guestrooms is uniquely decorated. Each also benefits from a private garden, a terrace with an outdoor hot tub, and dramatic views across the island wilderness. The ambience at Son Blanc is always relaxed and dreamy.

Operating from April to October, the retreat offers guests an ever-changing weekly program of wellness and recharging activities that include pottery workshops, yoga classes, forest bathing, and star gazing. Events are held in different locations around the property to encourage guests to foster a deep

OPPOSITE The original farmhouse was faithfully restored using local rock, clay, sandstone, and limestone—materials that also feature largely in the internal renovations.

connection with their natural surroundings. As well as joining weekly group activities, visitors can also enjoy one-to-one treatments and private sessions that include holistic massage, oil facials, reflexology, Reiki, and Pilates. They are also welcome to participate in daily farming or gardening activities.

Beyond the farmhouse, beautifully landscaped gardens give way to farmland and open terrain, where guests have miles of trails to explore on foot or by bike, across open country or around the coastline, surrounded by flora and fauna. At mealtimes, they are treated to menus that draw on the simple, earthy, and generous local cuisine. Fresh, wild ingredients are cooked using traditional local methods such as smoking, chargrilling, pickling, or drying, and eaten communally, alfresco. ∗

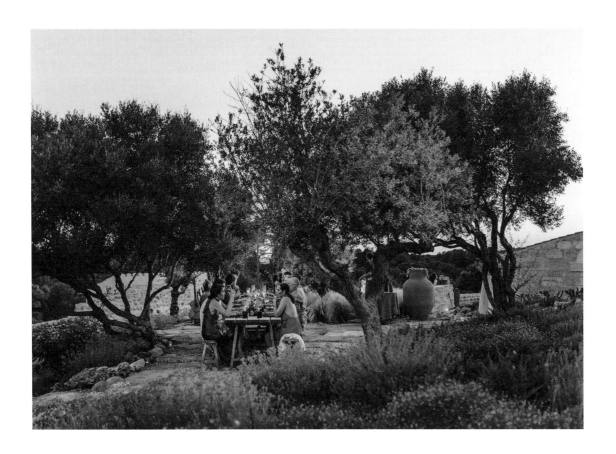

ABOVE AND OPPOSITE Bringing together local talents and inspiring visitors, Son Blanc Farmhouse's activity program maintains a balance of artist workshops, wellness therapies, and communal activities. It is inclusive and ever-changing throughout the seasons.

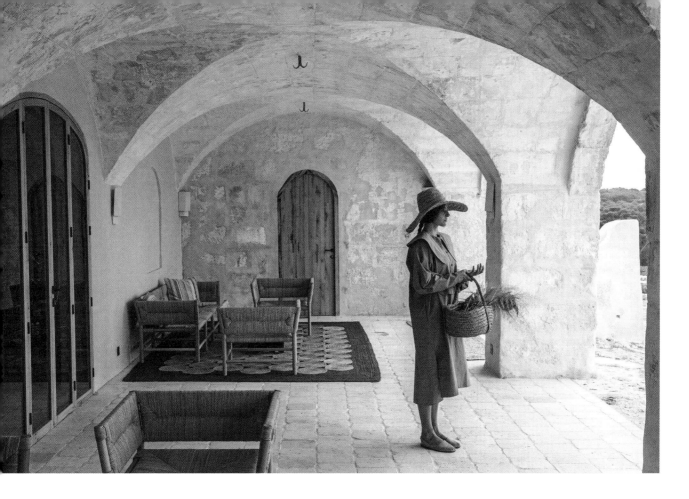

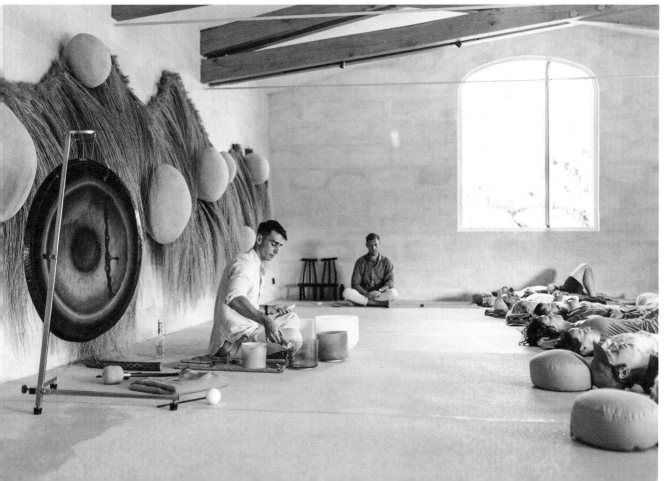

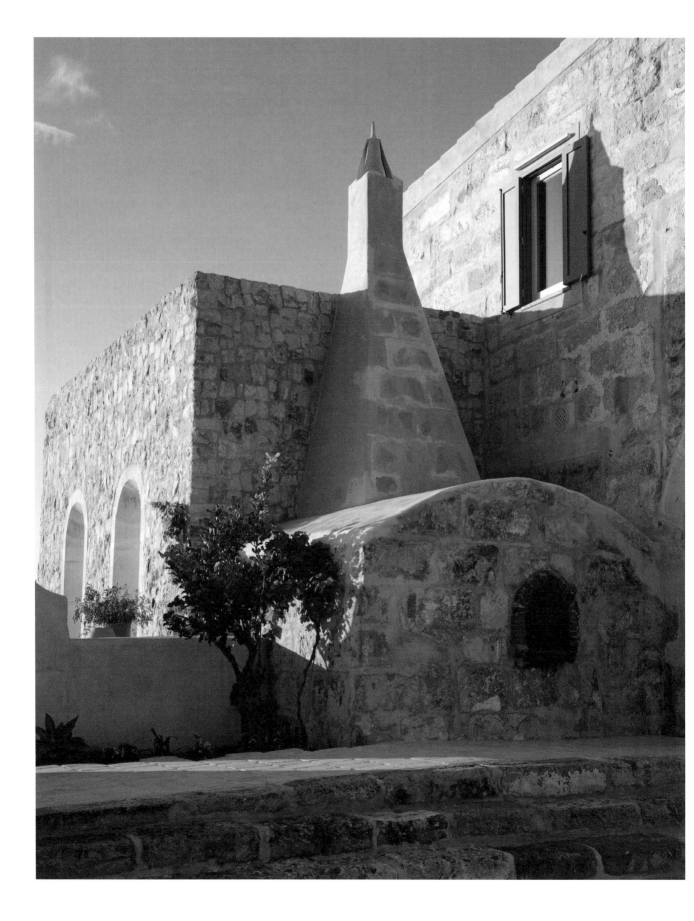

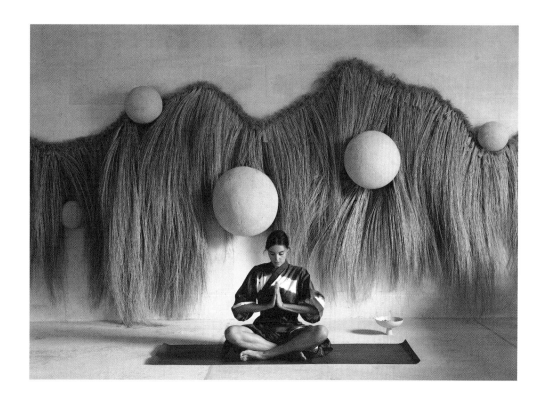

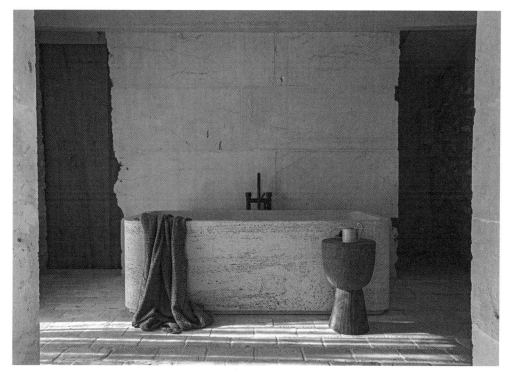

OPPOSITE AND ABOVE The resort is built around a collection of 19th-century farm buildings that were renovated and converted with great sensitivity, limiting their environmental impact through extensive use of local and natural materials.

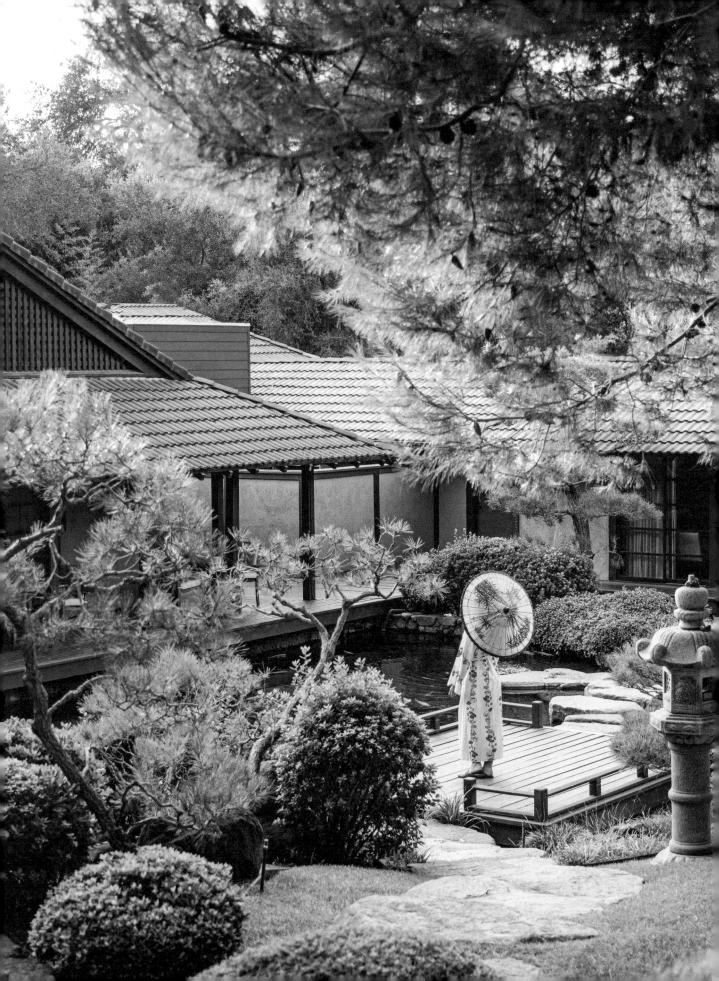

WHERE GUESTS EXPERIENCE THE LUXURY OF FINDING THEIR WAY BACK TO THEMSELVES

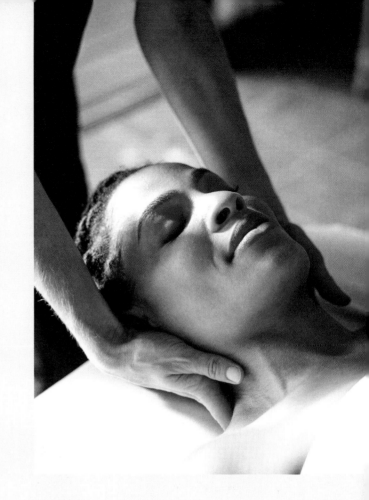

Golden Door
San Marcos, CA, USA

The Golden Door experience empowers guests to REPOSITION THEMSELVES at the center of their own lives by TENDING TO THEIR BODIES, their MINDS, and their SPIRITS via rejuvenating classes and luxury spa treatments.

According to the Golden Door philosophy, "a hike here is as much a rigorous morning exercise as it is a chance to reflect on the day ahead, and a meal is the means by which guests learn to satisfy rather than simply feed their hunger."

Located on 600 acres (240 hectares) of hills and meadows, with landscaped Japanese gardens, a citrus grove, and 5 acres (2 hectares) of bio-intensive gardens serving its restaurant, the resort in San Marcos, Southern California, is a luxury health retreat that few can rival. It offers guests 30 miles (50 km) of private trails, seven state-of-the-art gyms, two swimming pools, a *watsu* water therapy

pool, two labyrinths, tennis courts, pickleball, and a beautifully renovated bathhouse with a Jacuzzi, steam room, sauna, and nine skincare and body treatment rooms. A typical retreat package involves checking in on a Sunday for seven nights including a personalized program of healthy activities, holistic dining, and luxury spa treatments. All Golden Door guest rooms are single occupancy and have sliding doors that open onto a private outdoor patio with access to the beautifully landscaped Japanese gardens that lie at the heart of the complex. Warm-up clothes, T-shirts, and a bathrobe are supplied and laundered daily, and the owners also

OPPOSITE In the resort's Japanese gardens there are Zen rock areas for contemplation, quiet corners in which to drink tea, and *kaiyu-shiki-teien* gardens to stroll around.

supply a casual cotton kimono, sandals, Golden Door skincare products, a reusable water bottle, journal, tote, and yoga mat for guests' disposal.

During their stay, each visitor has an impressive range of activities to choose from, with four personal training sessions included in every retreat package. Classes that span yoga, meditation, and Pilates to fencing, swimming, cycling, rowing, and dancing take place in various venues inside and out. Classes dedicated specifically to mindfulness include haiku-writing, clay sculpting, and journaling. There are also sessions on pain management rooted in the practices of Feldenkrais and acupuncture, among others. Also included in each retreat package is a daily in-room massage from Monday to Saturday and five skincare sessions at the resort spa. Guests can indulge in one body treatment—a cherry blossom soak, a desert sea mud detoxifier, or a magnesium energizer, for example—two herbal wraps, a manicure, and a pedicure.

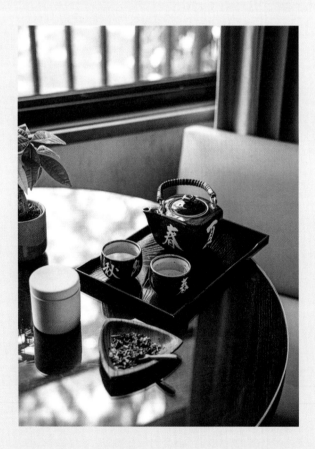

A hike here is as much a rigorous morning exercise as it is a chance to reflect on the day ahead.

ABOVE AND OPPOSITE The Japanese aesthetic runs throughout the resort—from its traditional tea-drinking paraphernalia to the *ryokan*-style architecture. Buildings are long and low with tiled roofs, dark-stained timber frames, and internal screens.

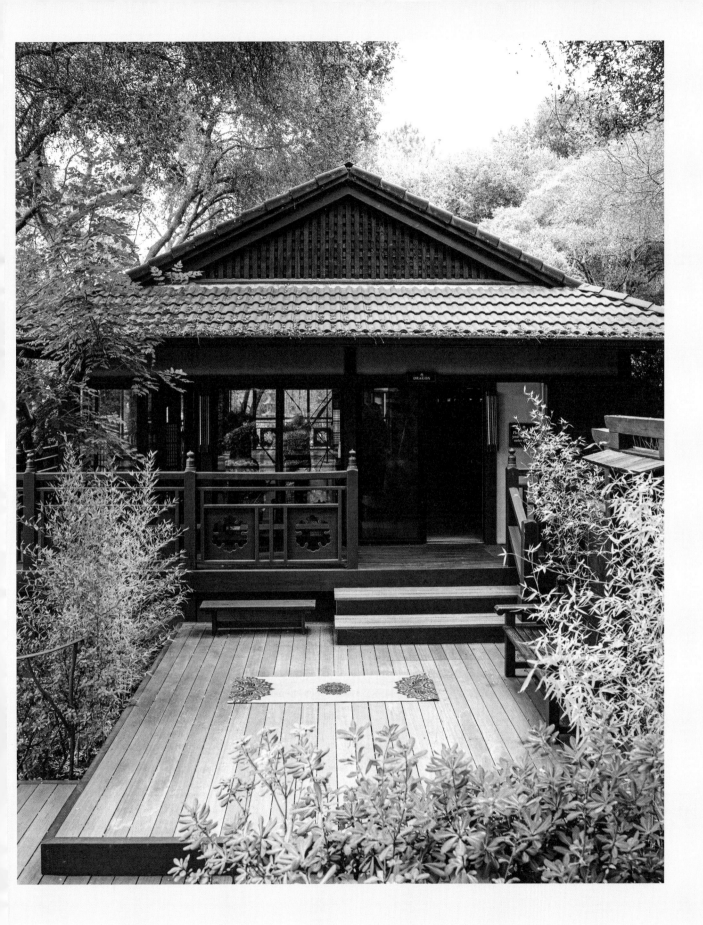

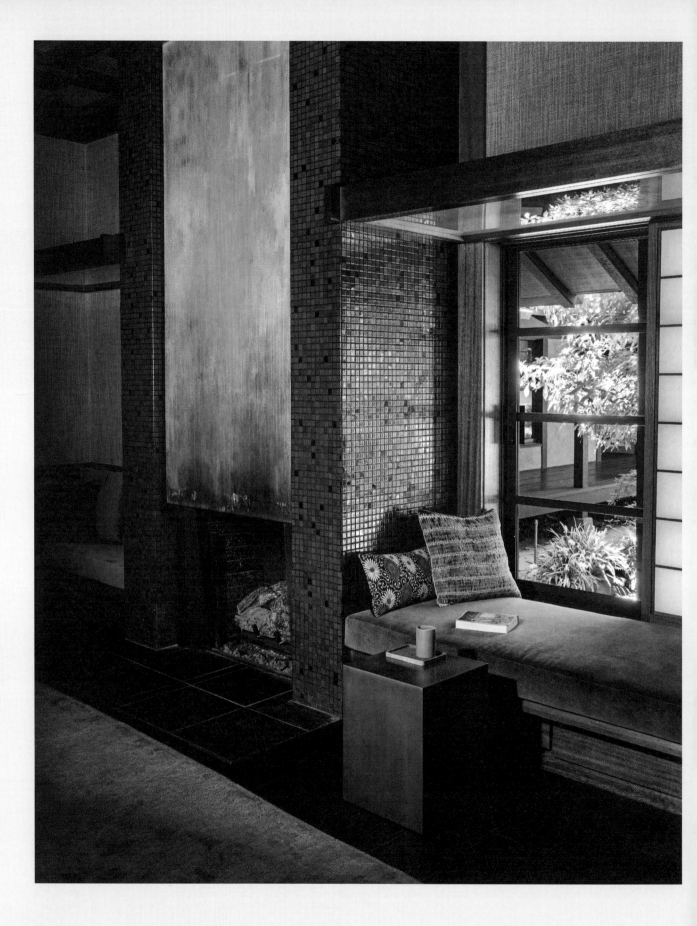

The resort's healthy food program includes meal plans designed specifically for each guest, focusing on fresh produce grown on the bio-intensive farm. On offer are three full meals a day plus mid-morning and mid-afternoon snacks, and appetizers before dinner. Guests can take part in a cooking class rooted in the resort's farm-to-table philosophy, and every stay includes an alfresco meal on the farm.

With each booking topped and tailed with courtesy transportation from San Diego or Los Angeles area airports, Golden Door really does offer the complete package. ✳

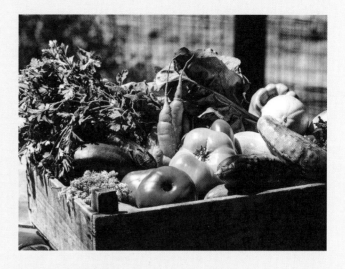

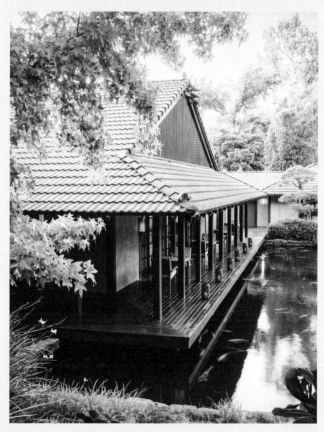

OPPOSITE The rooms at Golden Door are luxurious and stylish. Polished lacquered surfaces and mosaic tiling are juxtaposed with opaque screens and plush textiles in rich colors. TOP Meals consist primarily of organic fruit and vegetables grown at the resort's on-site bio-intensive farm.

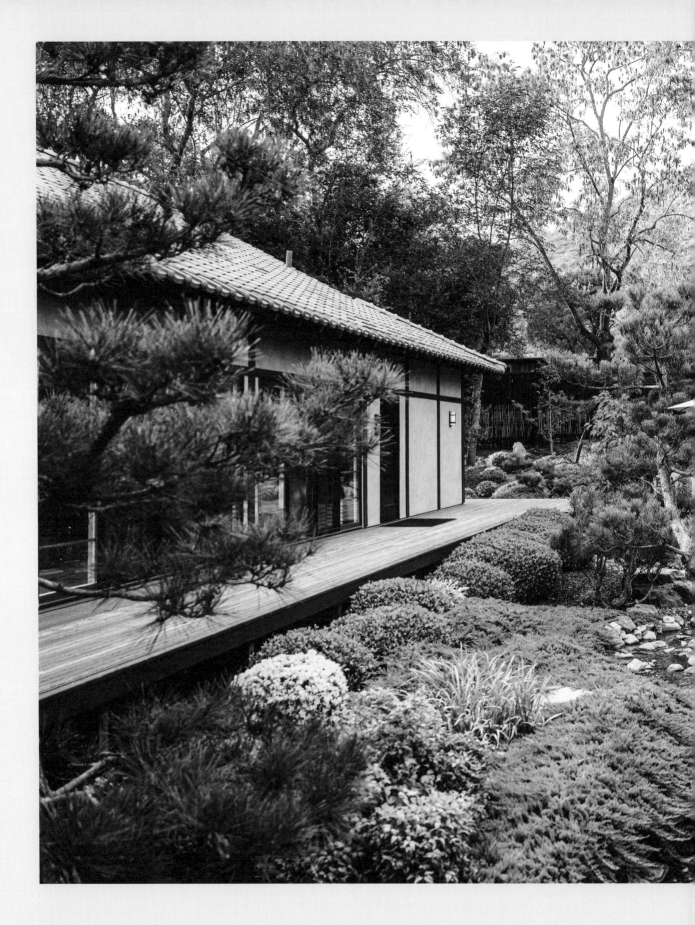

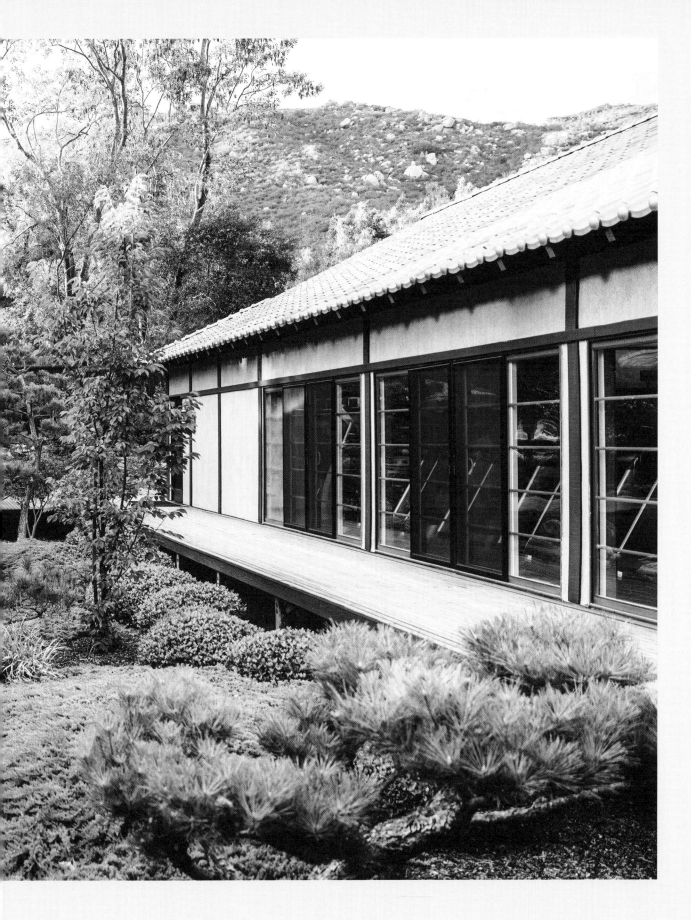

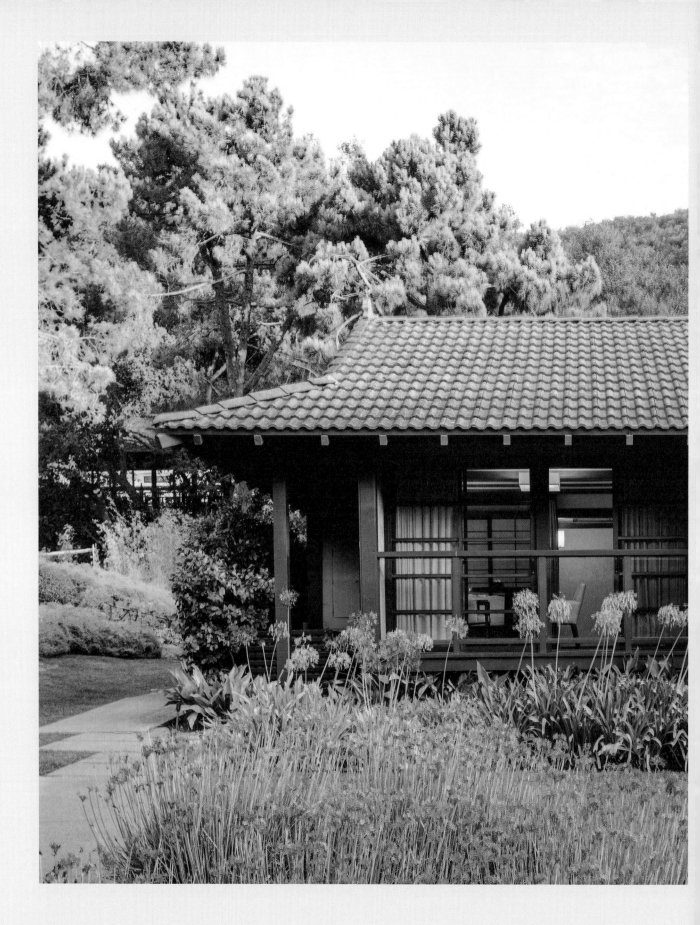

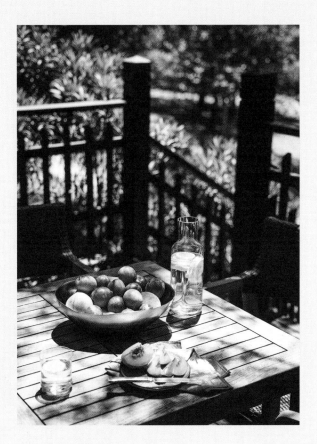

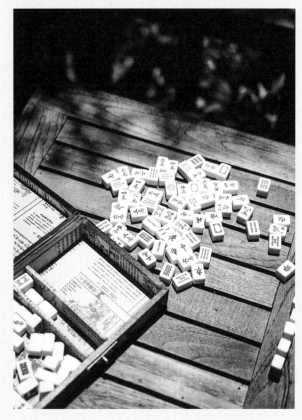

OPPOSITE Each of the guest rooms has its own private garden deck or patio space with access to the beautifully landscaped Japanese gardens. ABOVE There is an option to have in-room breakfast, and mid-morning snacks are available daily.

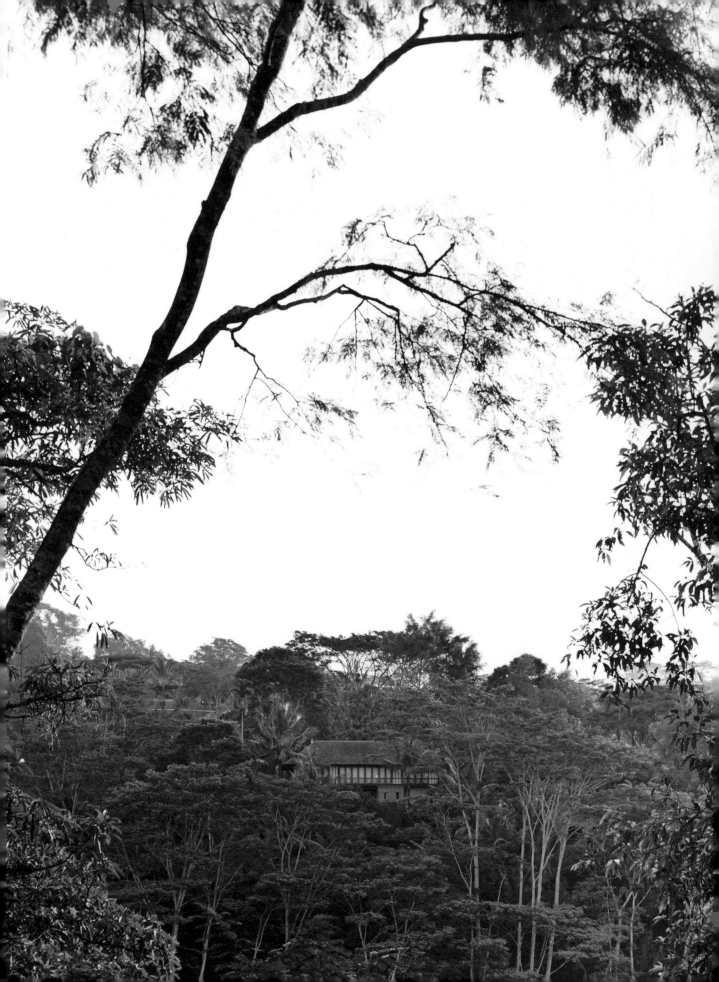

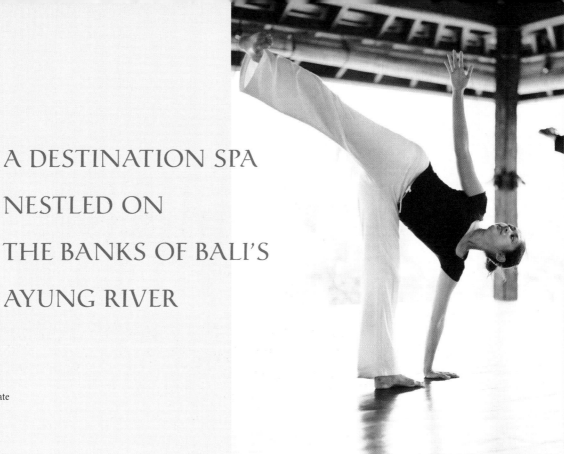

A DESTINATION SPA
NESTLED ON
THE BANKS OF BALI'S
AYUNG RIVER

COMO Shambhala Estate
Ubud, Bali, Indonesia

This wellness resort caters HOLISTICALLY *to the needs of each guest through tailored programs that combine* AYURVEDIC TREATMENTS *with outdoor activities and a nutritional food regime.*

The COMO Shambhala Estate is surrounded by lush forest on the banks of the Ayung River near the town of Ubud, in Bali. The retreat's architecture is inspired by the surrounding forest and the elements—wind, earth, fire, water—and draws on materials from the local environment. Buildings are made primarily from wood and stone and feature traditional Balinese *alang-alang* roofing, and each room is served with mineral water from a local spring.

Within the grounds are a host of amenities and facilities dedicated to well-being; they include a yoga pavilion, a Pilates studio, a vitality pool, and a gym. The resort also offers a wide range of holistic treatments—from massages, and bathing therapies to body wraps and facials—and specializes in a personal Integrated Wellness Program tailored to each guest's needs.

Guests at COMO Shambala Estate can choose from a range of accommodation, including several residences built in the middle of secluded forest and jungle clearings, with names like Forest in the Mist, Clear Water, and Windsong. These have rooms and suites alongside shared living spaces and a swimming pool and allow guests to fully immerse themselves in their natural surroundings. Those who prefer a more private experience

OPPOSITE The COMO Shambhala Estate is one of several COMO resorts around the world. Nestled in the Balinese jungle, it immerses guests in the sights and sounds of the forest.

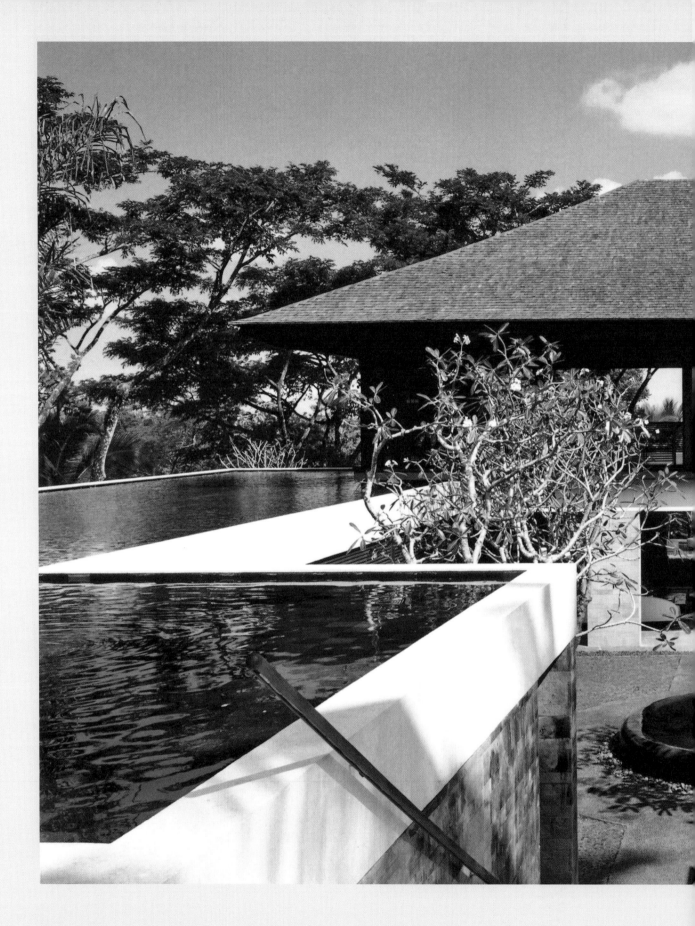

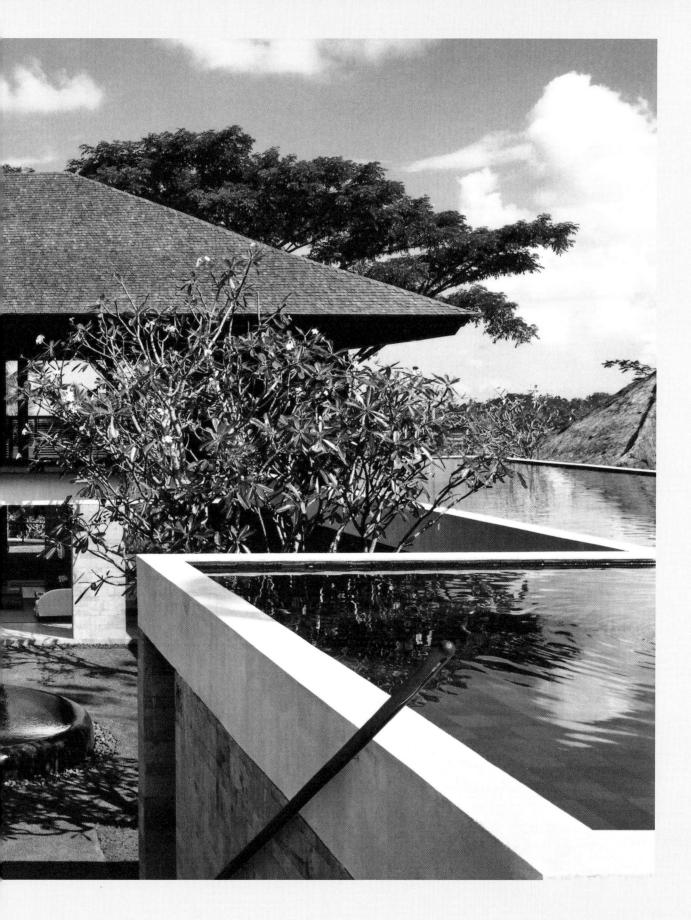

can rent a standalone villa with one to three bedrooms, a fully equipped kitchen and living room, and an outdoor terrace with swimming pool. No matter where they are on the estate, all rooms are tastefully furnished and have views across the forest as well as serene private spaces for quiet contemplation. When it comes to mealtimes, guests of the Balinese resort can choose from one of two on-site restaurants, Kudus and Glow, both of which serve well-balanced menus based on traditional Indonesian cuisine.

Glow is housed in a pavilion with views over the Ayung valley, while Kudus is set in a 19th-century Japanese villa. Guests can also choose from a healthy menu of snacks, granitas, and sorbets while at the Ojas spa or relaxing by the pool.

The popular Integrated Wellness Program offers a holistic approach in targeting a range of issues from stress to burnout to emotional fragility. During a seven-night stay (the minimum requirement for the tailored program) guests have a private consultation with a

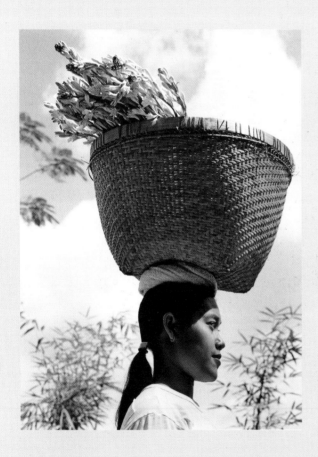

A personal assistant designs a daily routine, complete with a therapy schedule, eating plan, and wellness activities.

OPPOSITE *Shambhala,* meaning "peace" in Sanskrit, alludes to the resort's pursuit of balance on behalf of its guests. The retreat's approach to wellness is holistic, combining modern science with ancient practices to align mind, body, and spirit.

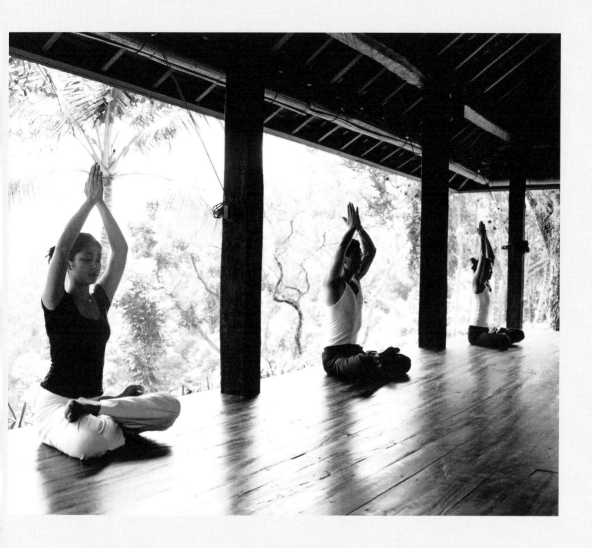

personal assistant who designs a daily routine for them, complete with a therapy schedule, eating plan, and wellness activities. Besides yoga, Pilates, and meditation classes, guests can take part in a diverse range of outdoor activities that include a rice field walk, a water spring blessing, a dawn ascent of local Mount Batur, and a purification ceremony. Back at the retreat, guests can indulge in relaxing massage and body care treatments, many of them with an Ayurvedic focus. All meals are included and carefully planned to suit the individual needs.

Bali enjoys a balmy year-round tropical climate with daytime temperatures in the area averaging around 80 °F (27 °C) and nights just a little cooler. The best time to visit Bali is May through to September when there's less humidity. ✳

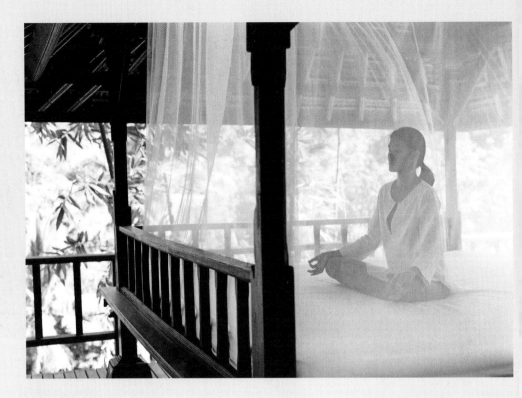

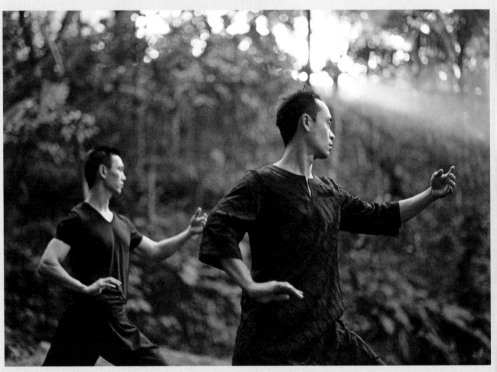

ABOVE AND OPPOSITE Making the most of Bali's year-round tropical climate, many of the facilities and private accommodation have rooms that are open to the elements. It means that guests can feel close to nature while taking part in individual or group fitness and meditation sessions.

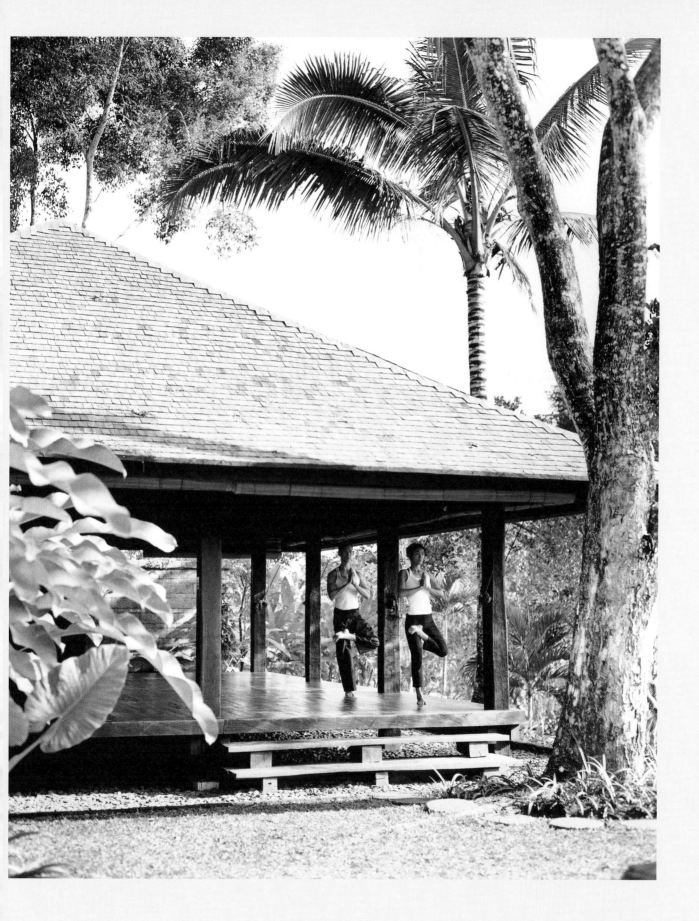

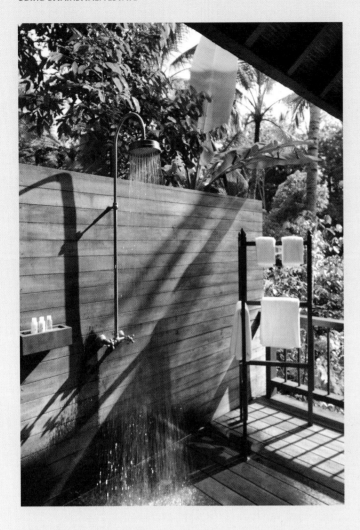

ABOVE AND OPPOSITE The resort was designed by architect Cheong Yew Kuan, who worked with interior designer Koichiro Ikebuchi. Though the end result is one of luxury and modernity, their vision reflects great respect for the local environment and the vernacular architectural style.

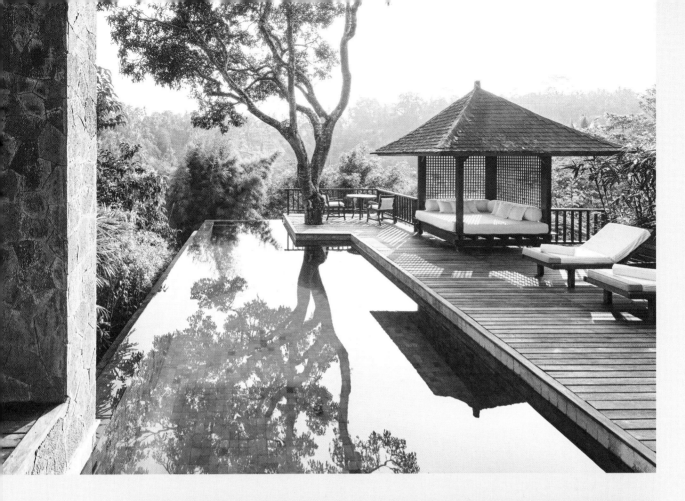
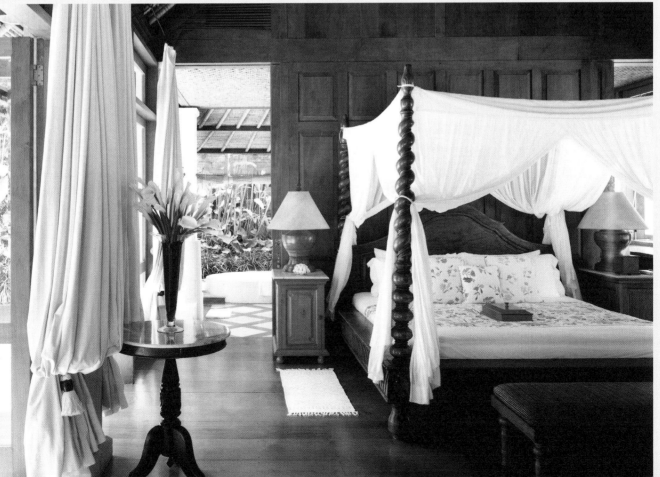

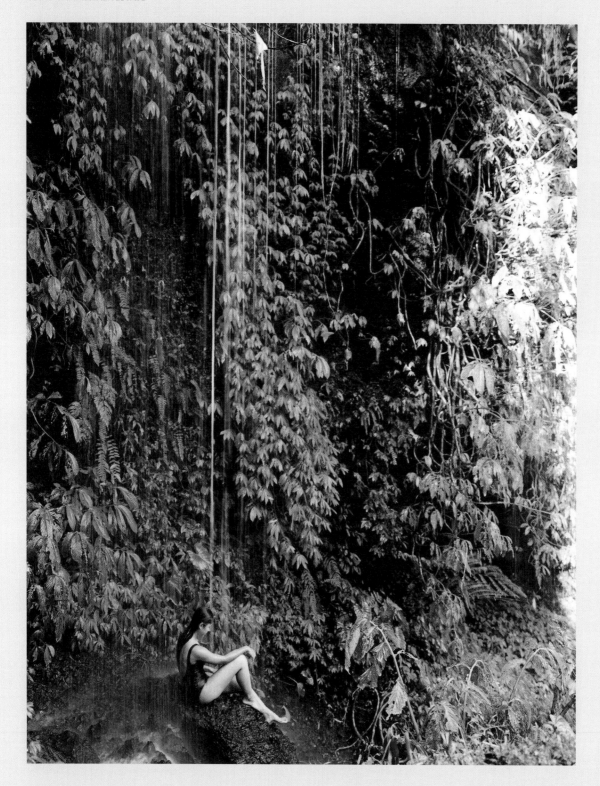

The architecture is inspired
by the forest and the elements—
wind, earth, fire, water.

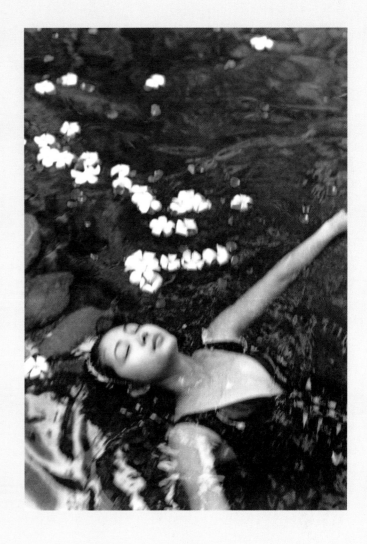

OPPOSITE AND ABOVE Besides the estate's own water-based activities, which include an outdoor vitality pool, private infinity pools, Jacuzzis, and a natural spring, there are countless natural pools and waterfalls on the grounds and in the forest beyond.

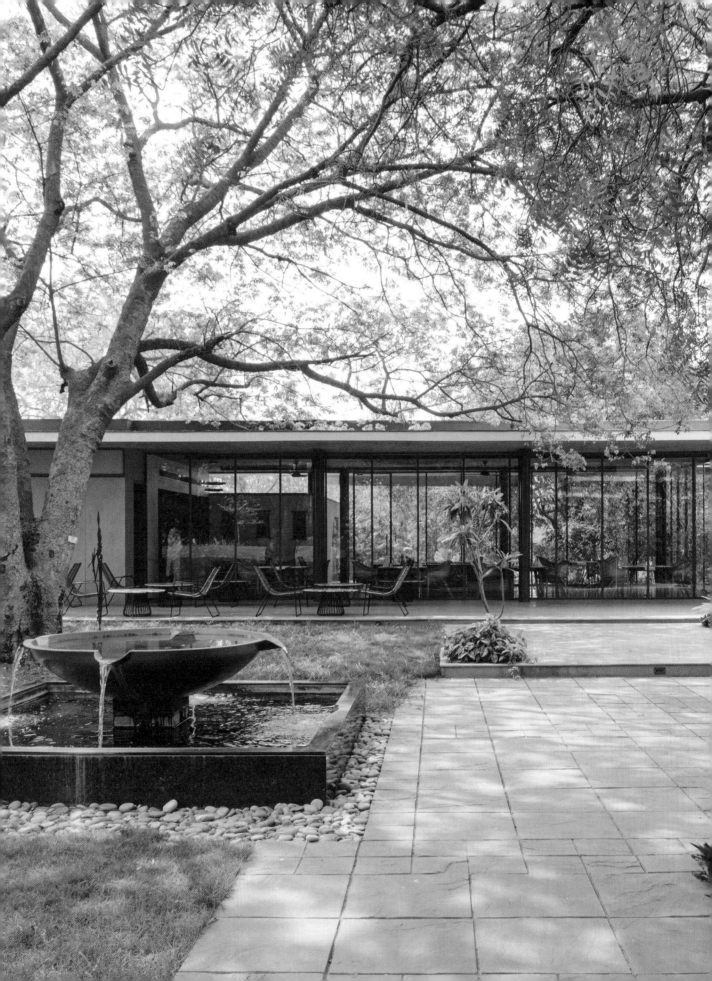

A SOULFUL JOURNEY TO SERENITY AND WELLNESS IN AN INDIAN OASIS OF PEACE

Raga Svara
Rajkot, India

With an emphasis on the ANCIENT THERAPIES and philosophies of Ayurveda and yoga, this retreat in India specializes in wellness programs that are TAILOR-MADE to each person's individual needs.

Serene and lush with foliage, the Raga Svara retreat is located in Rajkot, in the state of Gujarat in western India. The campus has been designed to ensure that there are plenty of private garden spaces and communal outdoor spaces, alongside fruit orchards and vegetable gardens. Such is the planting here that the grounds of the resort are beautiful throughout the year; the trees, plants, and flowers change dramatically throughout the seasons.

On arrival, guests are introduced to a personalized program based on their preselected retreat. Several options are available, among them a Wellness Retreat, a De-Stress Retreat, a Weight Management Retreat, and a Women's Health Retreat. Each has a set duration; the Wellness Retreat, for example, has a minimum of one night's stay, the De-Stress Retreat, five nights, and the Women's Health Retreat, seven. Each program blends the spiritual with the physical and includes a daily range of Ayurveda therapies, yoga classes, breathing techniques, and meditation sessions.

Also key to each tailor-made retreat at Raga Svara is a carefully curated, highly personalized dietary regime, based on seasonal ingredients, many of which are grown in the on-site garden. Organic spices and local and ecologically sustainable grains form the basis of many dishes. Guests are encouraged to practice mindful and slow eating to avoid overeating and to build a personal connection with the food.

Whether staying in a Megh Suite or a Raga Villa, guests are treated to spacious and luxuriously appointed rooms, each with an en suite bathroom and private outdoor space.

OPPOSITE The sleek modernist buildings at Raga Svara have the least possible impact on the natural landscape, which is populated with banyan and peepal trees.

BELOW AND RIGHT The retreat's ethos is to slow the mind and body via therapeutic treatments and meditation so that guests can properly connect with themselves and their surroundings.

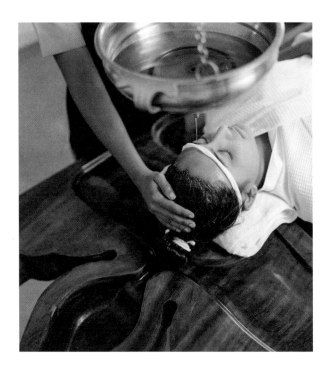

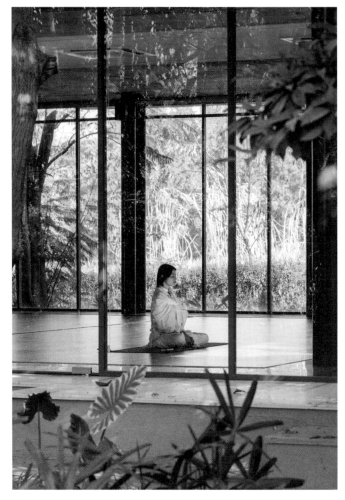

The villas also have their own plunge pools. Daily activities follow a rhythmic programming that changes with the seasons. Many are performed outdoors, where there is an overwhelming sense of living in harmony with the natural surroundings. The best times to visit are during the monsoon season (July to October) and the winter season (November to February) when daytime temperatures are more comfortable, although all indoor areas are centrally air-conditioned.

At the heart of an experience at Raga Svara is the owner's desire for guests to learn how to heal: "Our goal is to provide a holistic experience to rejuvenate the body and mind. It is about understanding, in totality, the wonderful tradition of health and wisdom, practicing, learning, and having a transformative experience." *

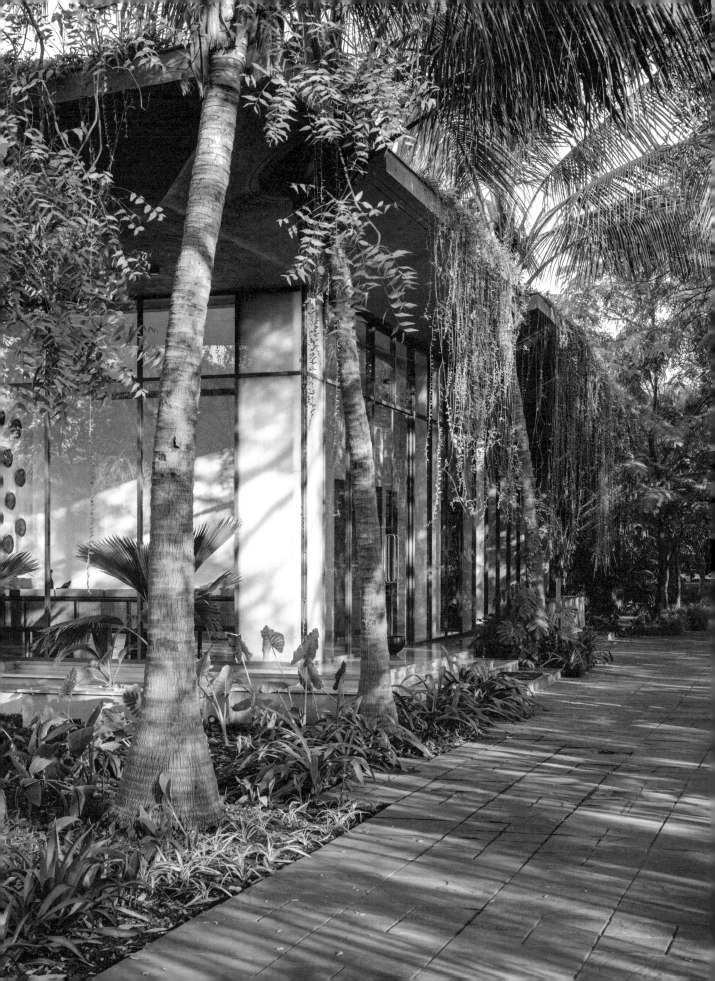

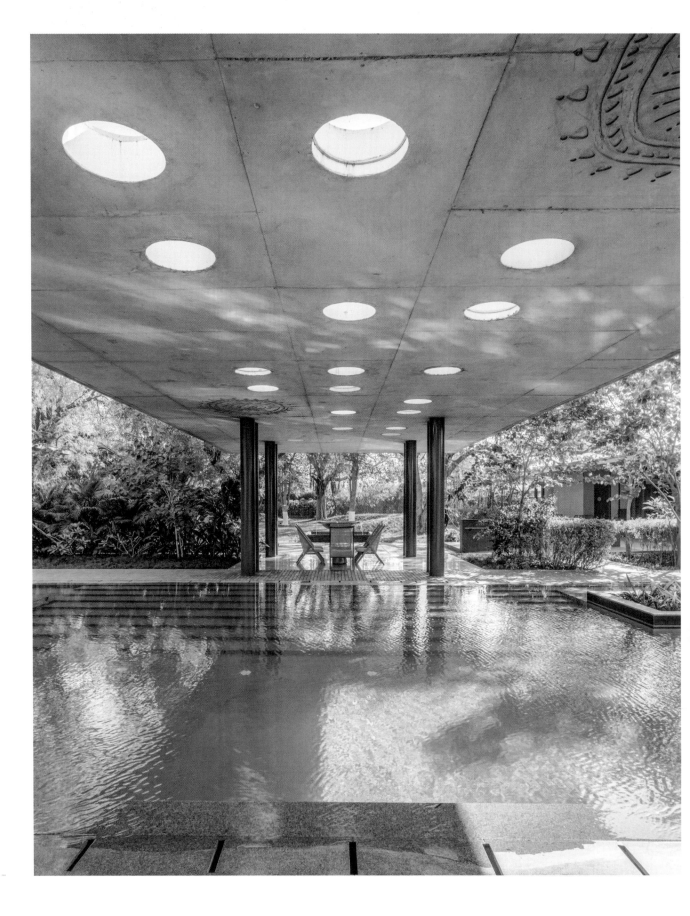

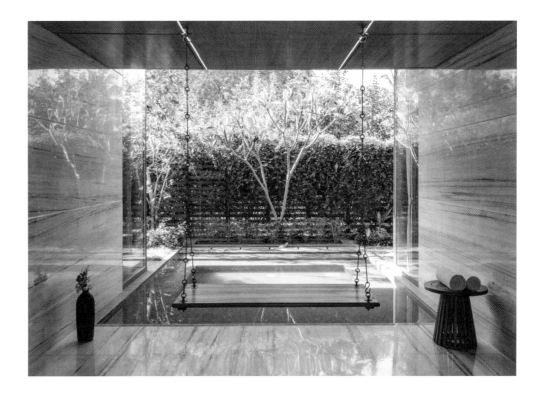

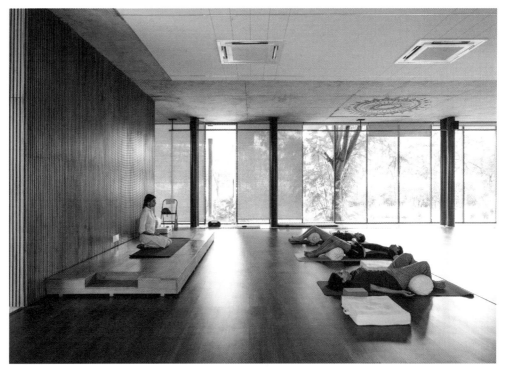

OPPOSITE At the heart of the campus is an inviting communal swimming pool that spans indoor and outdoor spaces, surrounded by lush vegetation. TOP Each guestroom also has its own private plunge pool for solitary bathing.

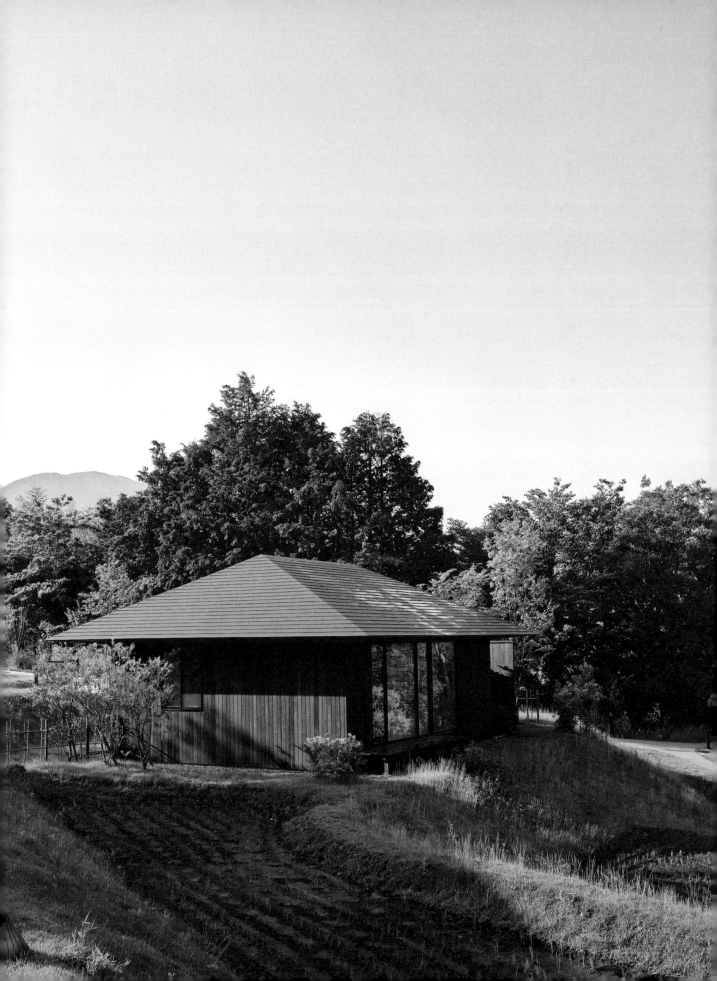

A TRADITIONAL JAPANESE-STYLE INN IN THE HOT SPRING TOWN OF YUFUIN ONSEN

KAI Yufuin Hoshino
Yufu, Japan

Set in a RURAL VILLAGE landscape in the Oita Prefecture of Japan's Kyushu island, guests find themselves bathing in hot, mineral-rich SPRING WATERS surrounded by rice terraces.

Dominating the skyline beyond this traditional Japanese inn, or *ryokan,* Mount Yufu rises above a landscape lush with cascading rice terraces. KAI Yufuin's grounds are also planted with rice, allowing guests to fully appreciate their surroundings and to fall into sync with nature's rhythm. Depending on the time of year, they may witness the reflection of the clear blue sky on the still waters before planting rice, the fresh green leaves that emerge just after sprouting, or the rich gold of the rice straw in fall. Possibly the best time to visit is September, when the rice terraces are lush and green.

With 45 rooms in total, accommodation is in the main building or in independent suites in the grounds. Guests can choose from six room types, all of which are decorated in simple, Japanese style, with a calming neutral palette and bamboo furnishings made by local craftspeople. In the Firefly Room a ceiling light hanging above the bed was inspired by the straw baskets once used to keep fireflies in as sources of light. The lamp casts a soft ambient light across the room that flickers slightly to evoke the movement of fireflies flitting about on warm summer nights.

For mealtimes, an on-site restaurant offers menus based on local and regional food. For dinner, for example, a multi-course *kaiseki* meal might feature a starter of wild boar meat and shitake mushroom pâté sandwiched in *monaka* wafers—a typical agricultural product of the Oita Prefecture—followed by a *shabu-shabu*-style hotpot of thinly sliced beef and game meat with a range of dipping sauces. While staying at the *ryokan,* guests can spend time relaxing in two indoor baths. The first,

OPPOSITE Built in the style of a traditional Japanese farmhouse, buildings at the retreat are long and low with spacious verandas overlooking the rice fields.

atsuyu (hot water), flows directly from the source, whereas the second, *nuruyu* (warm water), has a gentler warmth. An additional outdoor bath has a terrace on which to relax in the seasonal breeze after bathing. The spring water here is soft and rich in meta silicic acid, which is used in cosmetics as a skin conditioner, and bathing in it gently heals the mind and body.

The retreat offers a three-day itinerary that combines bathing sessions with breathing exercises, morning workouts, and neighborhood walks. Guests can also join traditional Japanese craft sessions and can book in-room therapeutic massages by nationally certified staff.   ✳

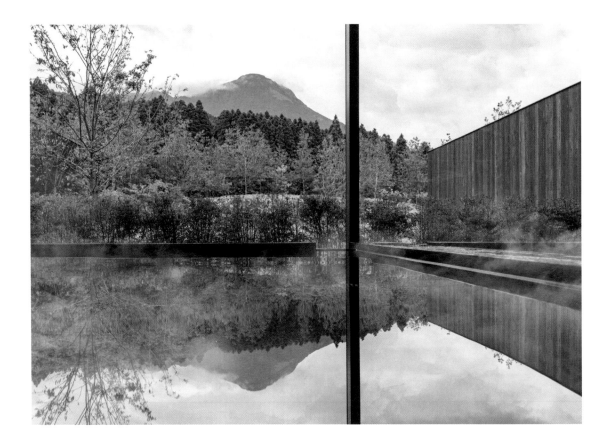

ABOVE The outdoor hot spring pool. OPPOSITE, TOP Guests can join a craft class, braiding straw into rope to create a traditional *oita* good luck charm. OPPOSITE, BOTTOM A typical *kaiseki* dinner, featuring seasonal ingredients and served in traditional *onta* ware.

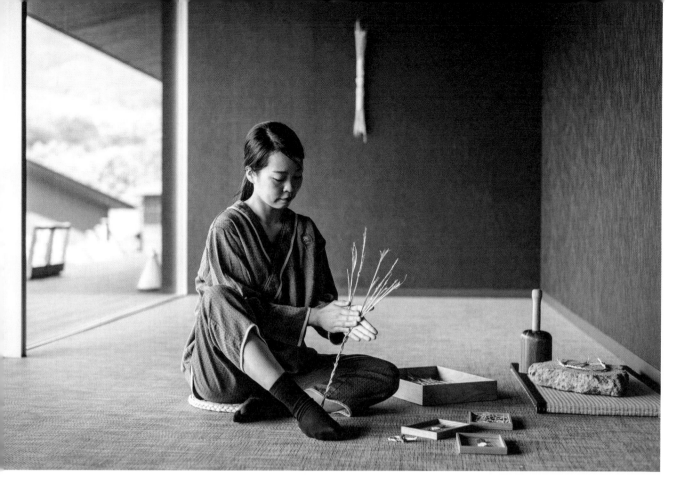

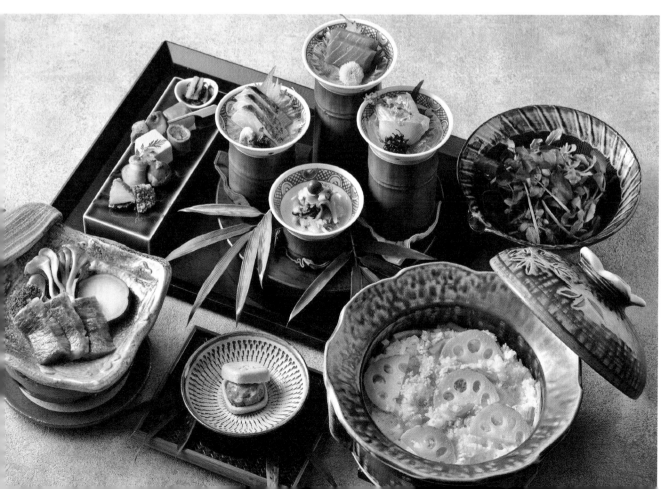

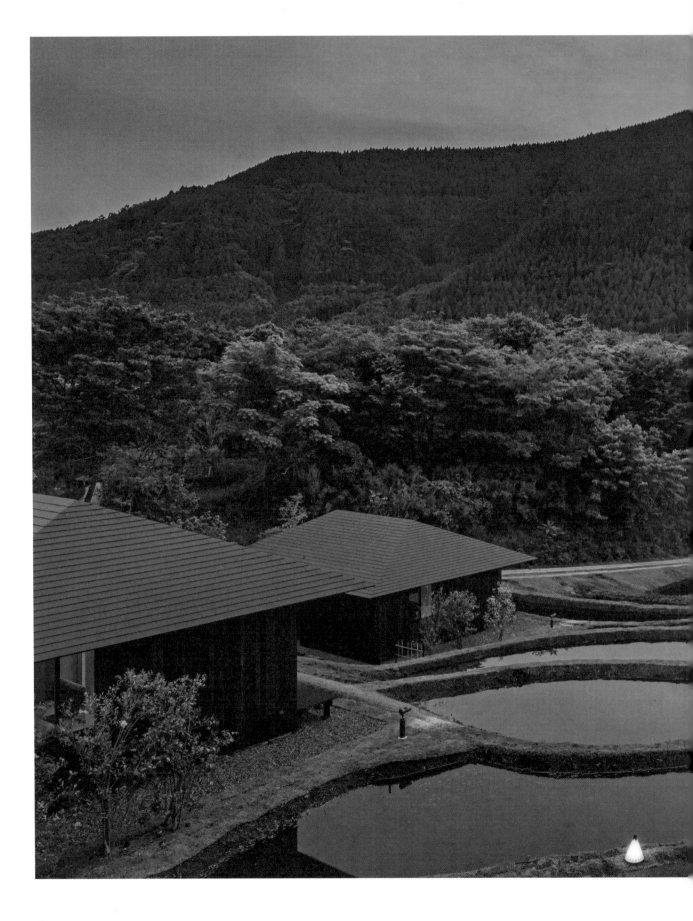

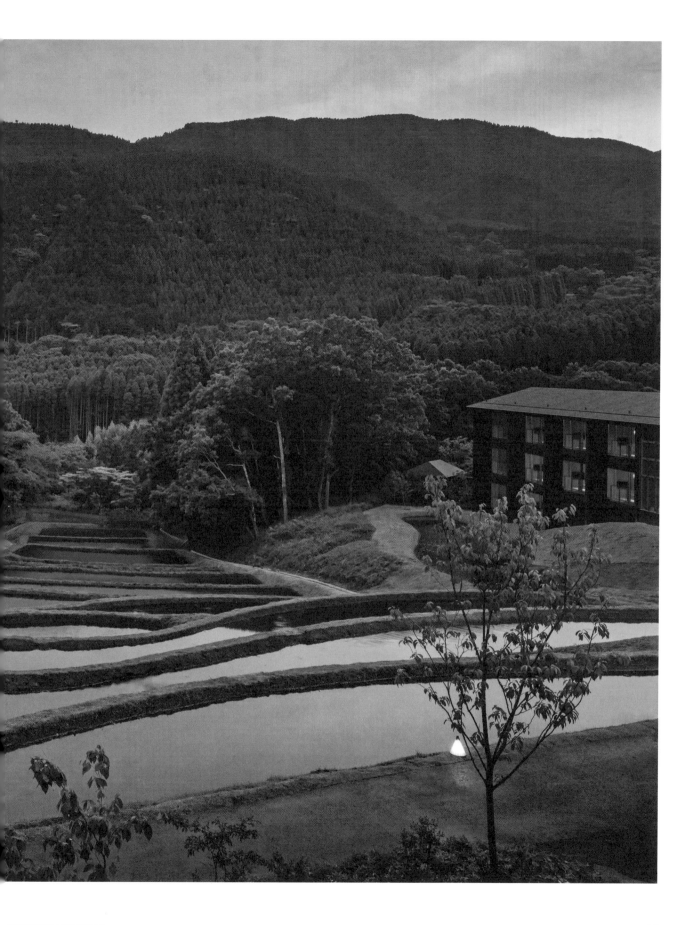

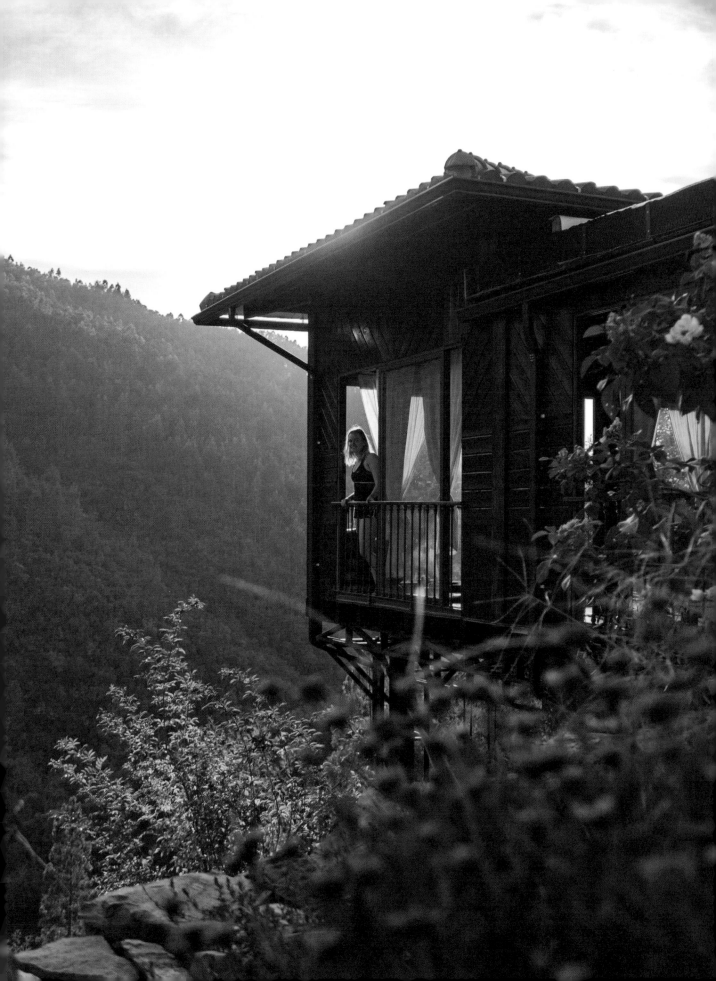

A MOUNTAIN RETREAT OFFERS
A HEALING, OUTDOOR YOGIC
WAY OF LIFE

Vale de Moses
Amieira, Portugal

Following the contours of a forested river valley, Vale de Moses is a peaceful yoga retreat that promotes TOTAL IMMERSION *in stunning natural surroundings while fostering* A DEEP SENSE OF COMMUNITY.

Every week, guests at Vale de Moses come to this forest-edged valley in the mountains of central Portugal to join a yoga retreat like no other. Owned and run by a family with support from like-minded locals, there is an overwhelming sense of community as guests relax and revitalize via a well-considered program of shared activities and individual treatments.

Accommodation for up to 25 people is spread around the hillside property, where guests can choose between a private room in the main farmhouse, a shared, open-plan cottage in the river valley below, and one of the bell tents mounted on separate stone terraces beneath the shade of Medronheiro, or "strawberry," trees. Though simple and rustic, there is no shortage of comfort here. Rooms are fully furnished with carpets and high-quality bed linen and there are bathrobes and hot water bottles for cooler nights. Sustainability is paramount at Vale de Moses, and cottages are equipped with thermodynamically heated showers and dry compost toilets.

Guests are encouraged to spend almost all of their time outdoors, and hammocks, benches, and deck chairs are placed in nooks and crannies so they can sit, read, write, or nap in the stillness of the forest, surrounded only by the sounds of running water and birdsong. Once settled at the retreat, guests can choose from a daily menu of activities, largely dictated by their preferences. Group sessions and communal mealtimes are interspersed with individual treatments and free time for self-exploration.

The main focus at Vale de Moses is yoga. Each day of the retreat starts with a group

OPPOSITE Suspended above the valley, the retreat floats above the landscape, surrounded by the sounds of cascading waterfalls, birdsong, and leaves rustling in the breeze.

session in the wooden *shala* before breakfast and a selection of afternoon workshops on the yogic way of life ranges from guided meditations and yoga *nidra* to aromatherapy and *kirtan* (call-and-response chanting) in a large bamboo-covered space complete with fire pit.

In between, as well as taking the opportunity to immerse in the surrounding landscape—either hiking one of its many trails, wild swimming in its natural river pools, or relaxing in the domed poolside sweat lodge—guests can indulge in treatments administered by the retreat's therapists, experts in acupuncture, *tui na* massage, and energy healing.

Three times a day, everyone comes together to enjoy a communal meal made according to the principles of Ayurveda. A vegetarian/vegan menu, rich in pulses and grains, focuses on fresh vegetables, salads, and fruit from local producers. ✳

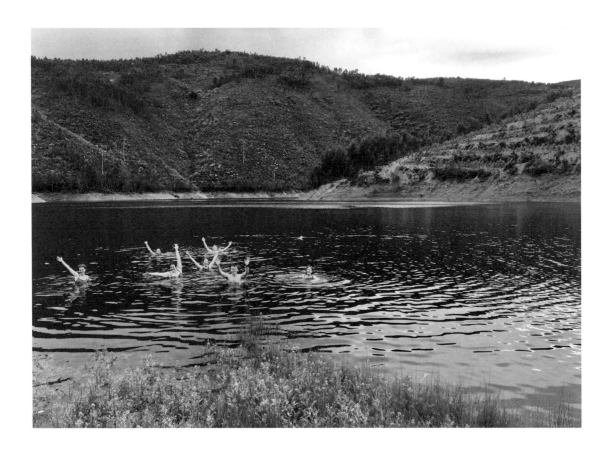

OPPOSITE The Xisto cottages at Vale de Moses was restored with great care and respect, adhering to local building traditions and using natural materials such as clay, lime, stone, and wood. They have wood-burning stoves, dry compost toilets, and thermodynamic or solar-heated outdoor showers.

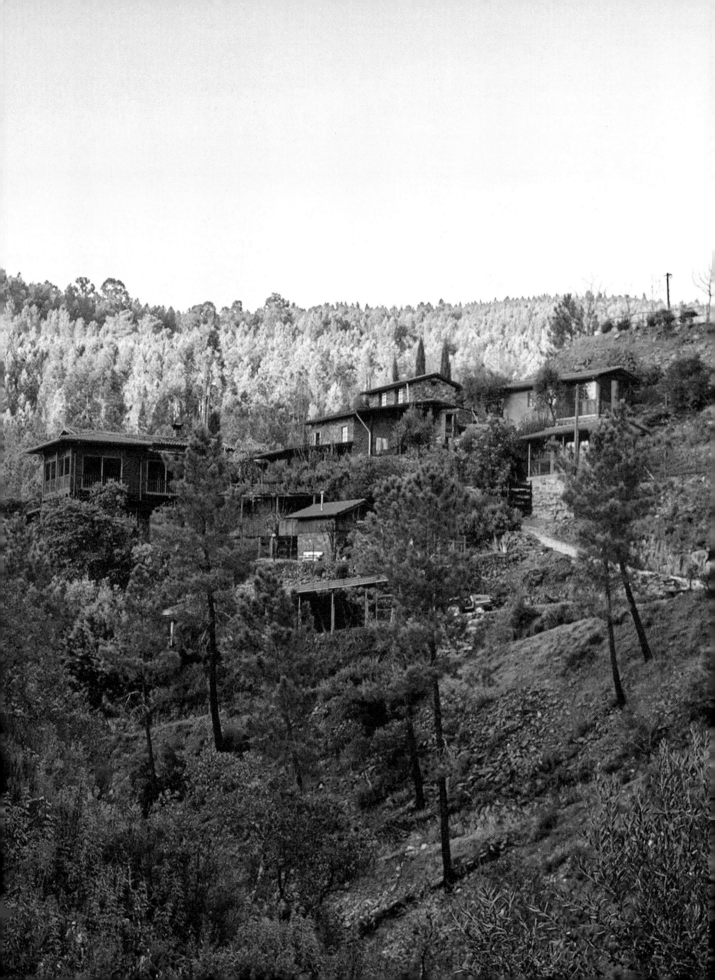

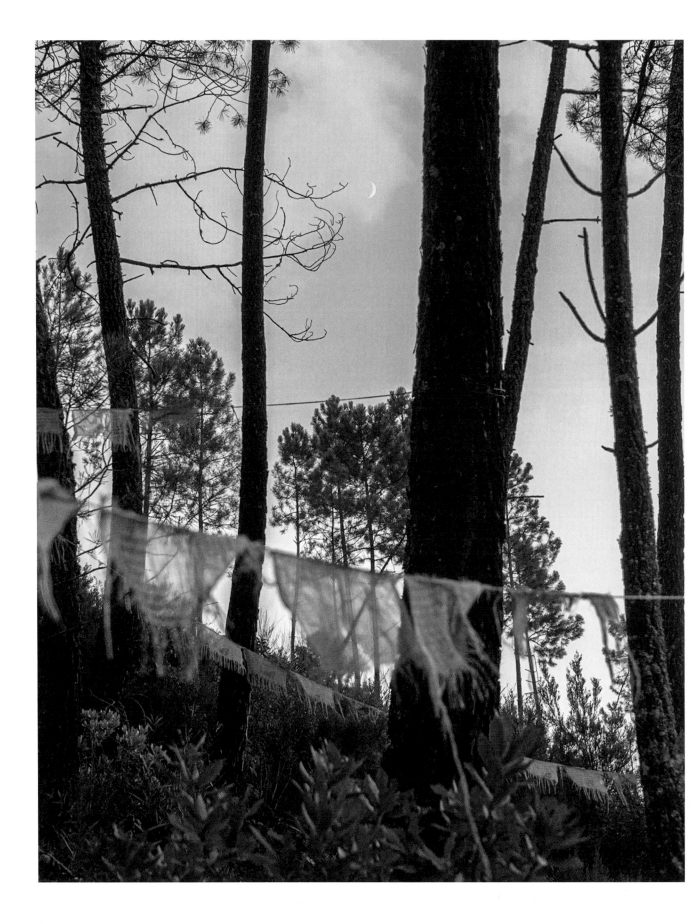

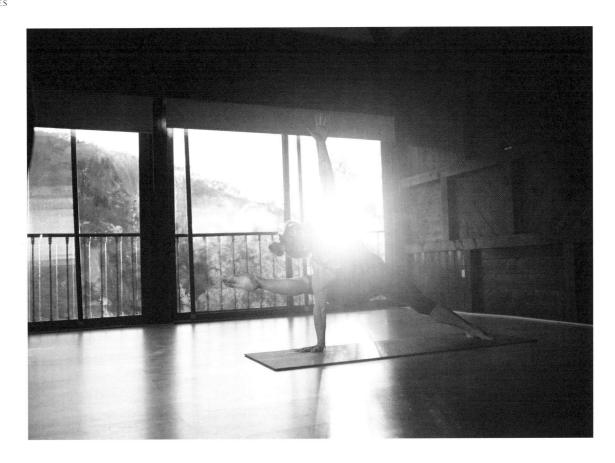

ABOVE Yoga classes are led by experienced practitioners and vary from flowing and energetic styles inspired by ashtanga, vinyasa, and dynamic hatha yoga to yin yoga, focused *asana* exploration, playful partner yoga, and quiet contemplation.

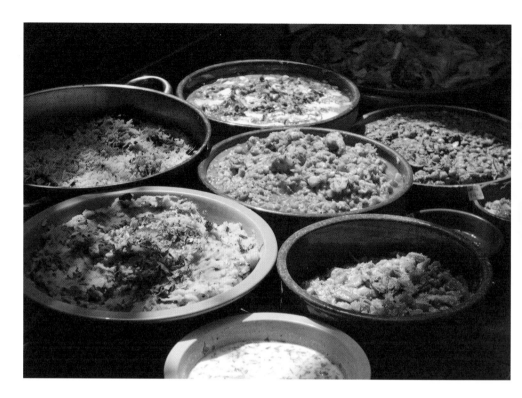

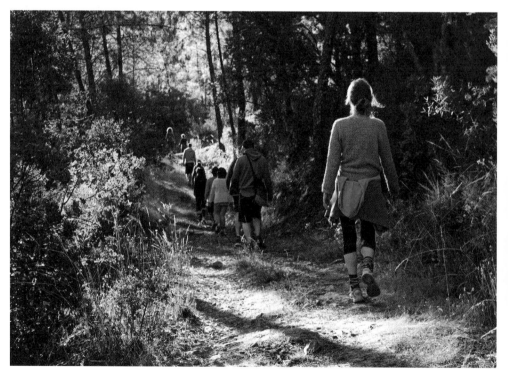

TOP Chefs at the retreat offer plant-based vegetarian and vegan food inspired by cuisines from all over the world—a fusion of ingredients, spices, and flavors. Prepared according to the principles of Ayurveda, every dish at Vale de Moses is not only tasty but also easy to digest.

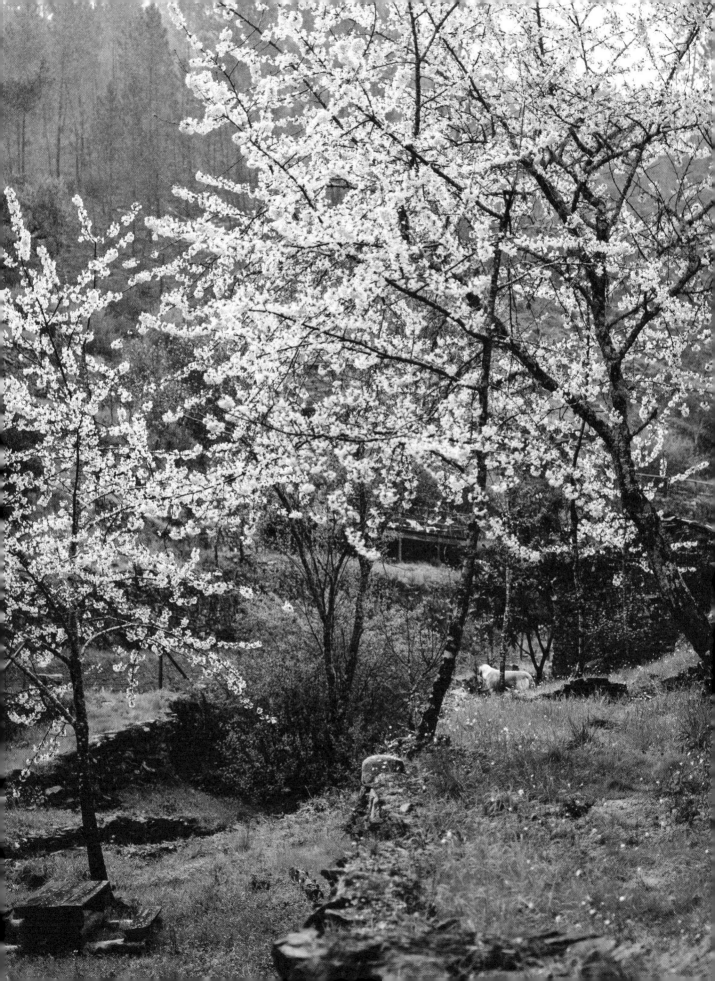

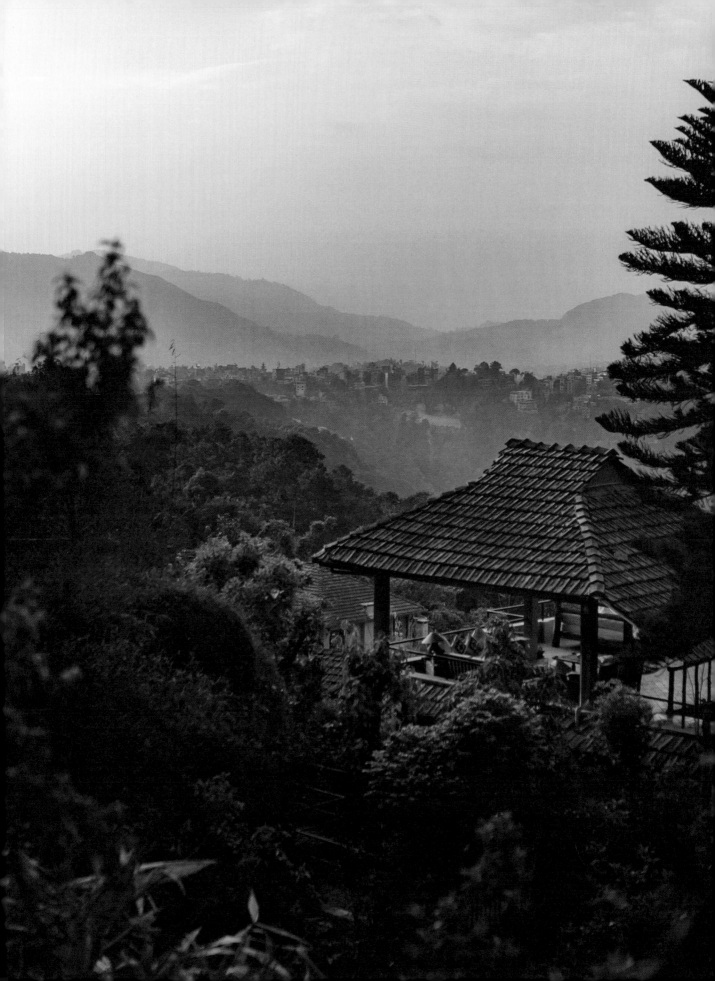

ENGAGING ALL FIVE SENSES TO REACH A STATE OF HARMONY AND REJUVENATION

The Dwarika's Resort
Dhulikhel, Nepal

A retreat in the foothills of the Himalayas, where guests explore a wide range of treatments and activities designed to achieve a PERFECT BALANCE *of mind, body, and spirit.*

A short drive from Kathmandu airport, the Dwarika's Resort is surrounded by woodland in one of the most serene landscapes of Nepal, with breathtaking views of the Kathmandu Valley and the Himalayas. With practices rooted in ancient Hindu scriptures, Buddhist medicine, and traditional Himalayan wisdom, the resort is built upon a philosophy that reveres nature and seeks to nurture harmony of the mind, body, and spirit. Central to a stay at the resort are activities designed to address each of the five senses and guide guests through their own personal journeys.

Guests are encouraged to stay a minimum of five days to benefit fully from the resort's offerings. There are 40 spacious suites with amenities that include en suite bathrooms, indoor and outdoor living spaces, and a private kitchen, all beautifully furnished and with luxury fittings and fixtures.

Included in the room price is an impressive range of facilities and activities such as unlimited use of the resort's meditation maze, a chakra sound therapy chamber, indoor and outdoor swimming pools, a sauna, and a hot tub. Guests are also entitled to a group yoga class and a communal meditation session, among other daily activities.

For a more structured retreat, or one dedicated to specific needs, the resort also offers a series of packages that include a Yoga Package, a Revitalization Package, a Revival and Relaxation Package, and a Cleansing Package. Lasting from four to eleven days, each package features a daily program of treatments and activities, starting with a private consultation with the resort's Ayurvedic

OPPOSITE Set on the slopes of the Dhulikhel hills in Nepal, the villas at the resort were built using traditional methods so that they blend in naturally with the landscape.

doctor. As an example of the kinds of therapies guests can expect, the Rejuvenation Package includes a stress-relieving massage, an herbal bath, a Himalayan singing bowl therapy session, a steam bath, and a hot stone therapy session.

All meals are included at the Dwarika's Resort and are centered on organic food from the resort's own farms. The overriding food principle here is "fresh, local, organic, seasonal, and less traveled." Meals incorporate key principles of Ayurveda and Buddhist cuisine, which take into consideration not just the taste of the food, but also its suitability for the body type. A meal here celebrates the origins of the food and is designed to nurture body, mind, and soul. *

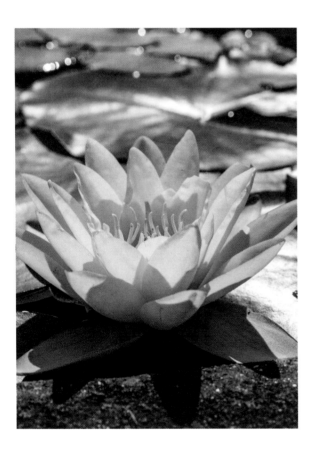

OPPOSITE At the highest point of the property—up among the treetops—the Ping terrace is an idyllic spot to take in the incredible beauty of the Himalayan landscape. Among other highlights for relaxation are the retreat's infinity pool and a meditation maze.

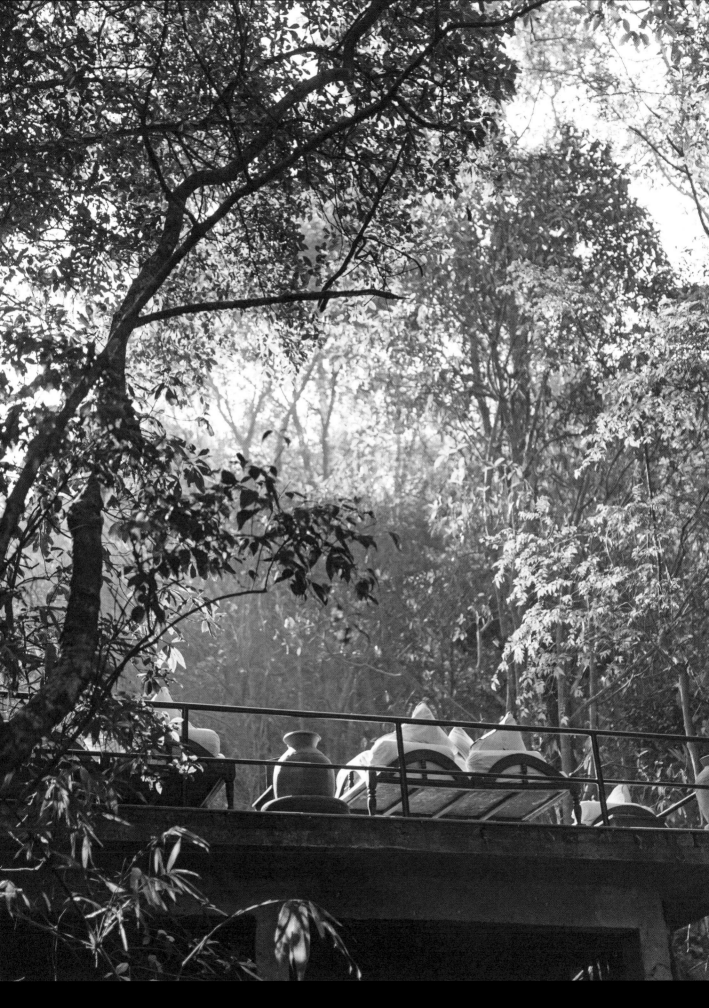

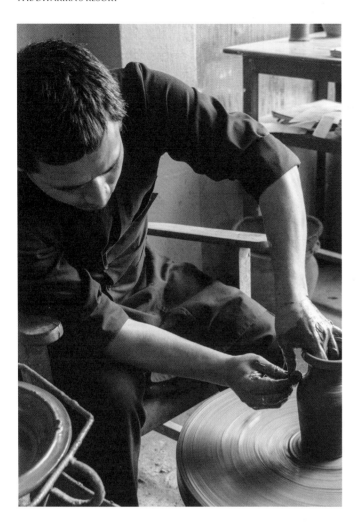

OPPOSITE, TOP The guests' suites integrate indoor and outdoor living spaces overlooking a dreamy landscape of forests and mountains. Each has its own character and is furnished with natural local fabrics in soft, warm, earthy colors to match those of the surroundings.

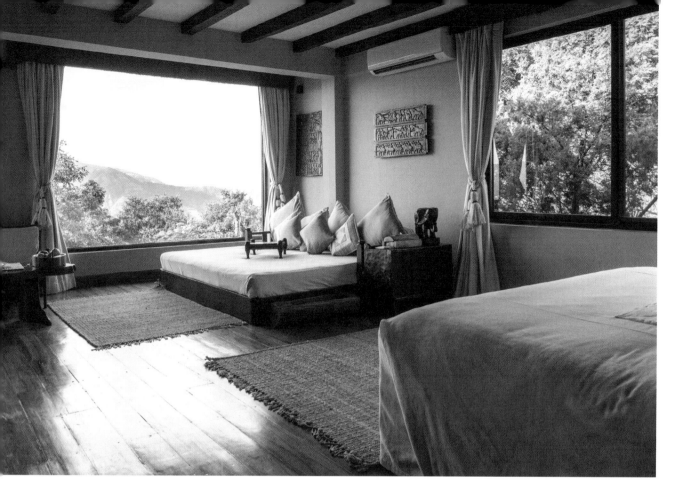
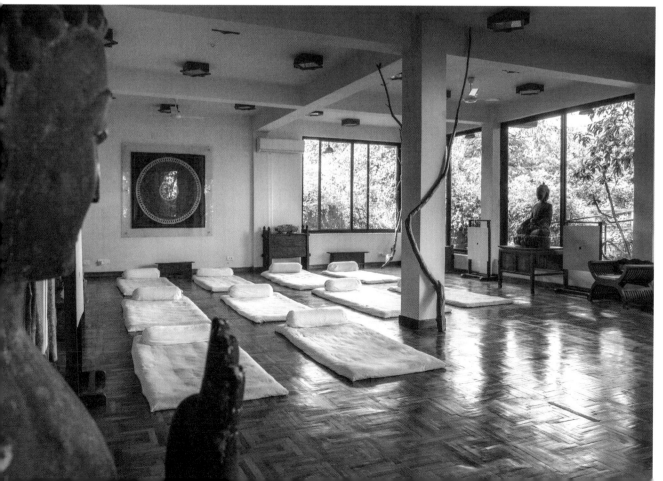

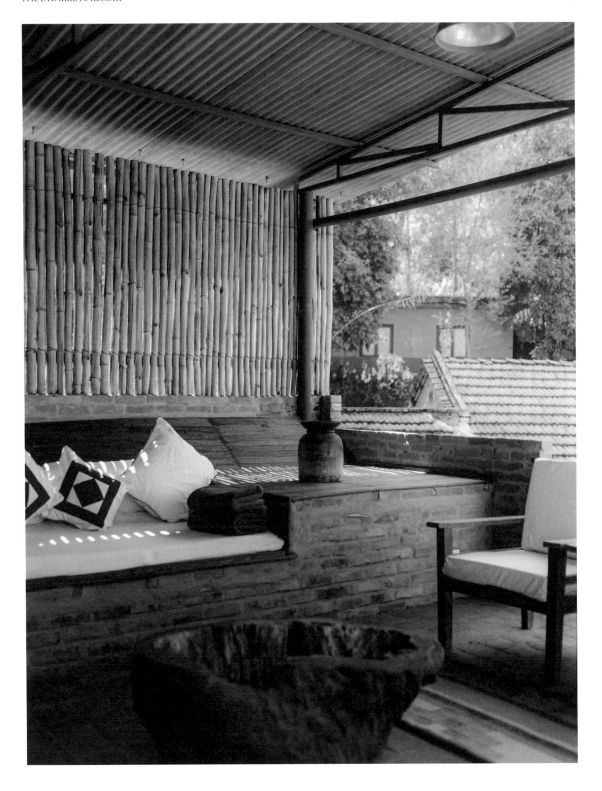

ABOVE A treatment room at the retreat's spa. The wide range of treatments on offer include Ayurvedic massage, hot stone therapy, and singing bowl therapy. OPPOSITE Stunning landscaped gardens offer guests numerous spaces in which to sit in quiet contemplation.

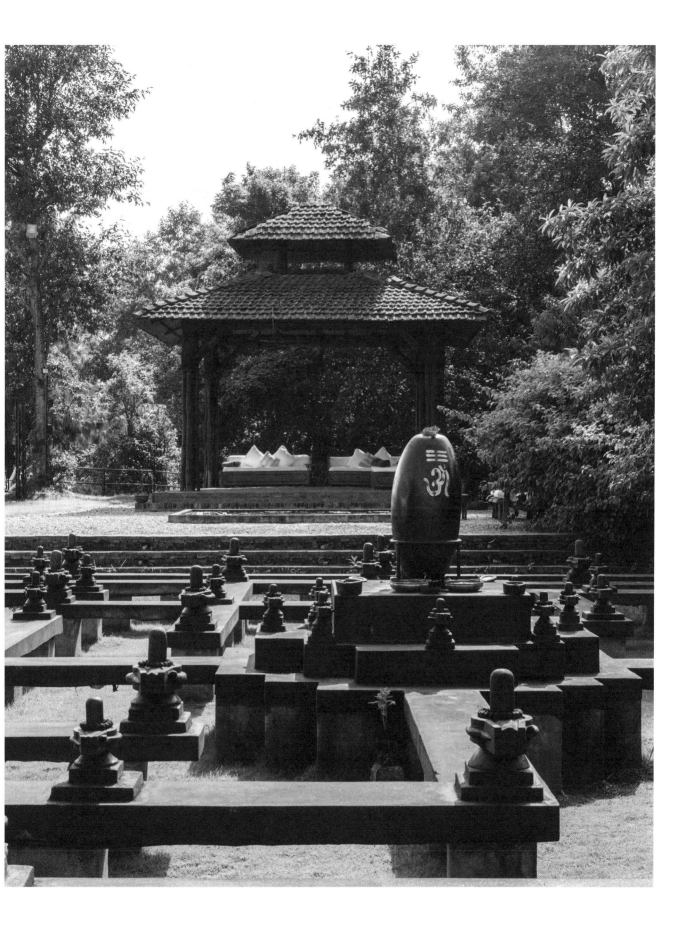

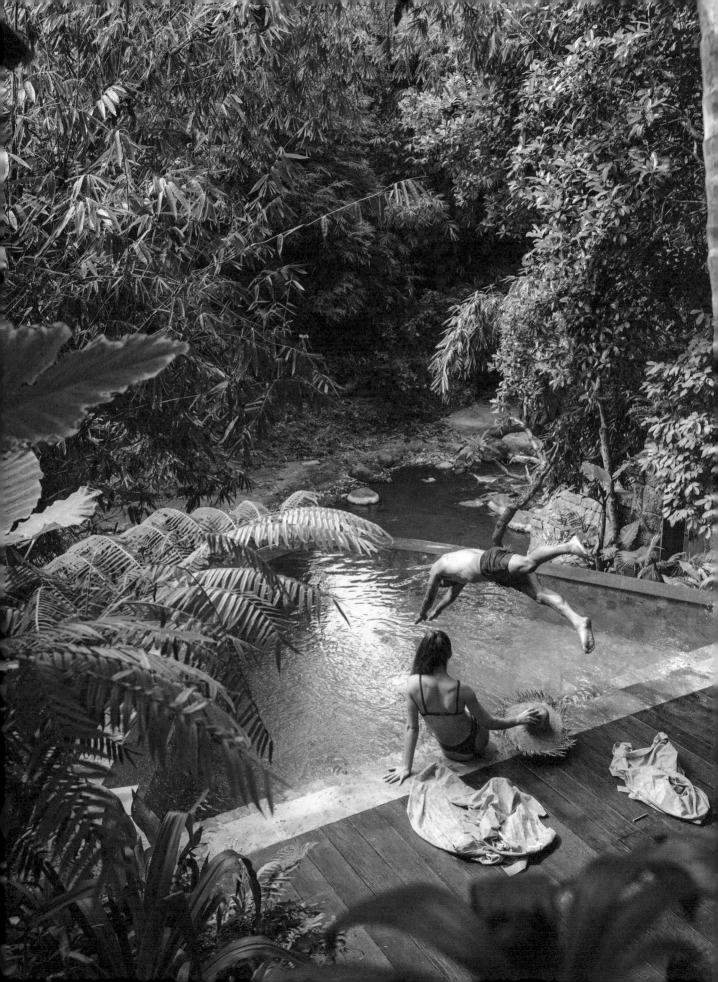

ULTIMATE RELAXATION AND REJUVENATION IN THE HEART OF THE BALINESE RAINFOREST

Suenyo Eco Retreat
Tabanan, Bali, Indonesia

Through TRADITIONAL HERBAL REMEDIES *and* REGIONAL CRAFTS *handed down through generations, guests find ancient* BALINESE WISDOM *woven into their every experience at this luxury island resort.*

Located just a 15 minutes' drive from the coastal resort of Canggu on the Indonesian island of Bali, this secluded retreat is surrounded by lush rainforest on the banks of the Yeh Poh River. Completely cut off from the modern world, it is the perfect setting to disconnect from the outside world and reconnect with the self.

The rich cultural heritage of Bali is a primary focus at the Suenyo Eco Retreat. Alongside the resort's wellness program, the retreat holds traditional ceremonies, such as the Balinese Melukat water cleansing ritual for spiritual purification, and runs workshops that celebrate artisanal Balinese crafts, from bamboo flute-making to lontar calligraphy led by master craftspeople. Meanwhile, the wellness program draws on the healing power of nature and traditional herbal remedies

in a range of massages, such as the signature Balinese Harmony Massage, and wellness rituals, such as the Divine Rejuvenation Ritual. Additional extras on the spa menu include a volcanic body mask, a foot reflexology session, an organic body exfoliation, and deeply relaxing flower or coconut milk baths. Guests can also join group yoga and meditation sessions in the riverside *shala*.

While staying at the resort, guests sleep in one of six exquisite bamboo pavilions designed with great care and consciousness to provide intimate, secluded, peaceful spaces for introspection and physical healing. Inspired by sacred geometry and the inherent strength of the parabolic curve, each pavilion is a series of organic, curved structures built from bamboo. Almost interwoven with the jungle canopy, the structures blend into their

OPPOSITE The spa facilities blend in seamlessly with the retreat's natural surroundings so that guests feel totally immersed in nature throughout their stay.

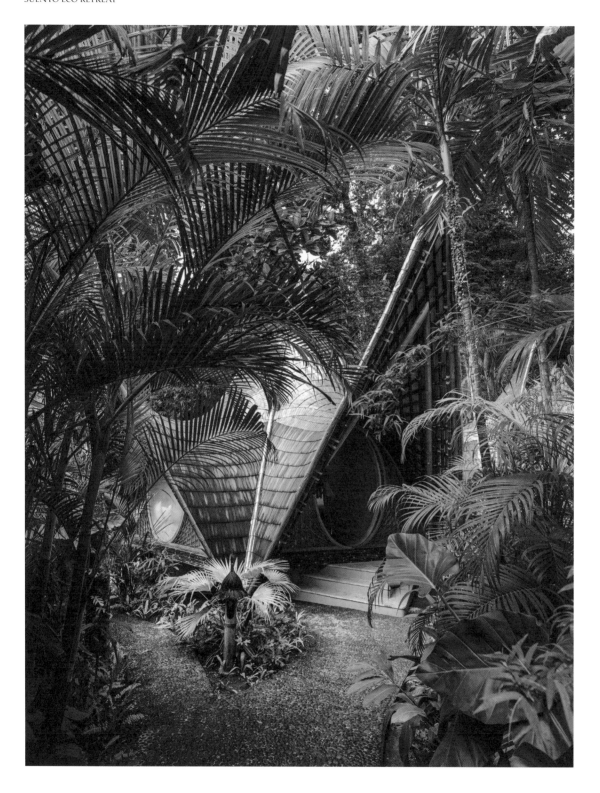

ABOVE AND OPPOSITE The resort's bamboo pavilions are works of art in their own right—stunning structures with mesmerizing curved walls and ceilings, oval windows and beds, and nets in which to stargaze. The pavilions vary in size and shape, the largest being a two-story, two-bedroom villa.

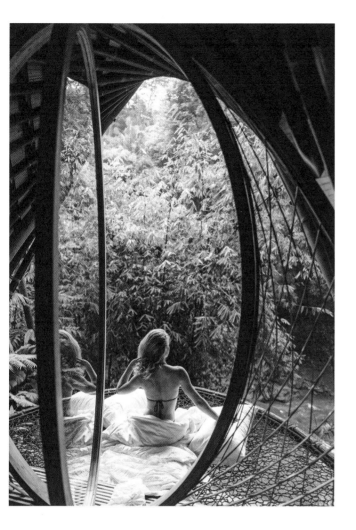

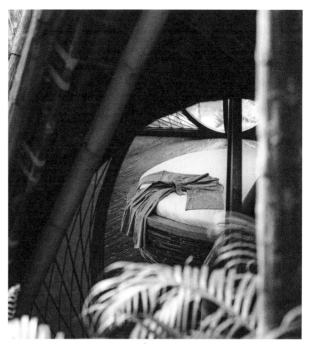

natural surroundings to create a magical atmosphere across the resort. Each one has a private deck with a suspended relaxation net, a stone bathtub, and an infinity pool.

The resort's restaurant makes the most of locally available ingredients, sourced from organic farms, and prepared in a refined, modern way. Menus are built around traditional Indonesian dishes that represent the rich cultural tapestry of the region—Pangsit Udang, for example, is a shrimp dumpling in a ginger flower bisque, or Nasi Bakar Jamur, mixed wild mushrooms with coconut rice and pickles. A minimum stay at the Suenyo Eco Retreat is two nights, but a trip lasting three or four nights would allow guests to immerse themselves fully in the experience of this beautiful luxury resort. *

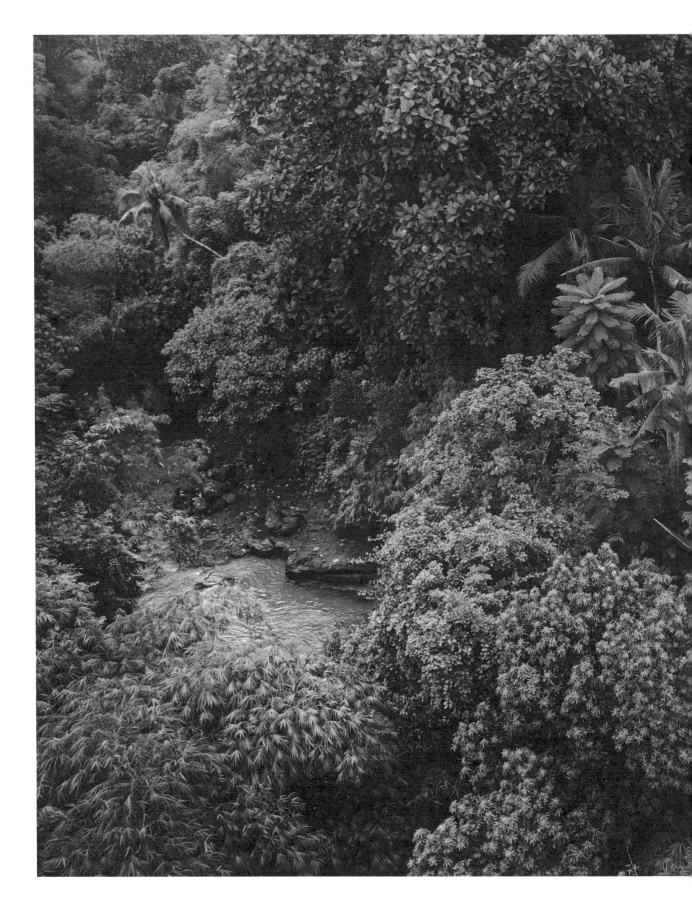

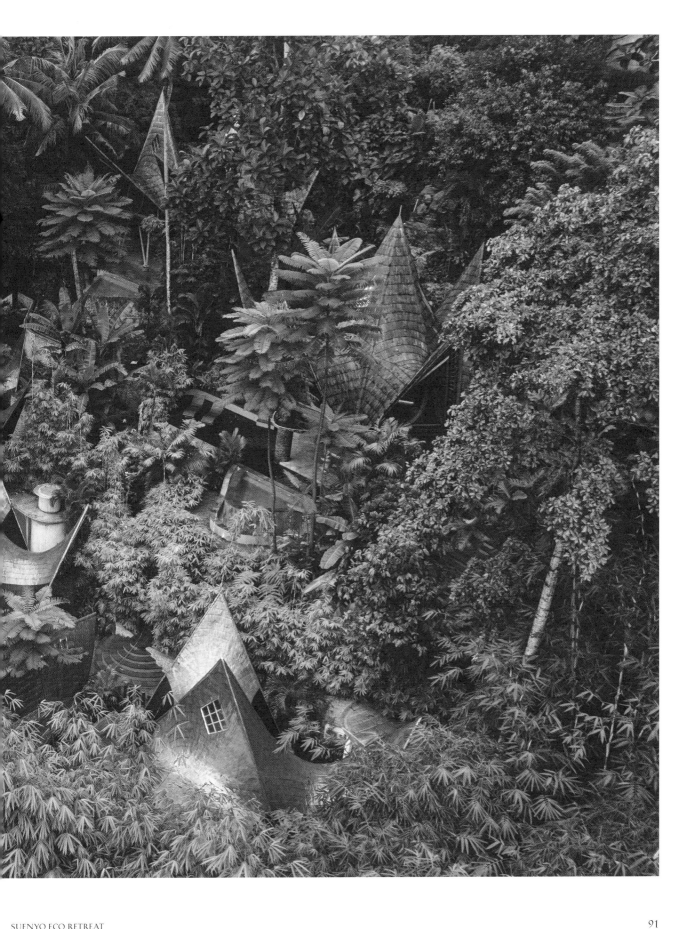

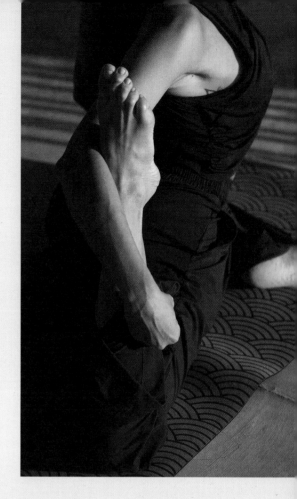

A FUSION OF WELLNESS AND LUXURY, THIS ISLAND ODYSSEY NOURISHES YOUR SOUL

EcoHotel El Agua
Arico el Nuevo, Tenerife, Spain

A sensitively restored 200-year-old BODEGA AND FINCA *offers a boutique bolthole for a tranquil Tenerife escape—the perfect backdrop for a range of intensive, transformative wellness programs.*

At the secluded, idyllic EcoHotel El Agua on the island of Tenerife, retreat founder Anthony Picq promises the resort's guests "gorgeous panoramic views, exquisite 'zero miles' dining, and nourishing holistic treatments."

Nestled in the historic, low-key village of Arico el Nuevo in a subtropical valley in the south of the island, the hotel was once crumbling farmland and is now a sanctuary for the body and soul. This lovingly restored high-end, low-impact retreat offers guests the benefits of holistic medicine in an environment surrounded by natural beauty. Guests are invited to come here to chill, recharge,

and disconnect, and they find themselves deeply reconnected with themselves by the end of their stay.

Until recently, this health-focused hilltop hideaway had capacity for just two guests who were lavished with attention for the duration of their stay and treated to the most extraordinary fusion of wellness and luxury from a team dedicated solely to their needs. Guests staying in the Villa Olivo, a cozy little stone house originally used as a winery, enjoyed complete solitude among the estate's olive groves. The formula has proved so successful that the hotel has since expanded to host up to 25 guests in a range of villas and

OPPOSITE Once a refuge for peasants who worked the land cultivating vines, this sun-blessed corner of a hilltop village is an oasis of peace and serenity.

suites both across the estate and in the village, treated with the same level of attention from staff. All the accommodation is stocked with top-quality organic bathing products and sophisticated entertainment systems for rest and relaxation, and receive a daily basket of organic fruit. All have access to private terraces and heated saltwater infinity pools. An expert in Hippocratic medicine, Picq's ethos at his retreat is to provide an "enchanting haven" for his guests, and "the ultimate oasis of wellness and creativity." To this end, he has devised four transformative wellness programs for guests to embark upon during their stay. Among these, the Detoxification and Regeneration program is based on internal cleansing and metabolic balance and includes intermittent fasting, a raw-food diet, and a daily massage. The Water for Health program is based on hydrotherapy with a daily breathing session, cold bath, and *watsu* massage session, among other treatments. Other programs focus on yoga activities and personal training/weight management.

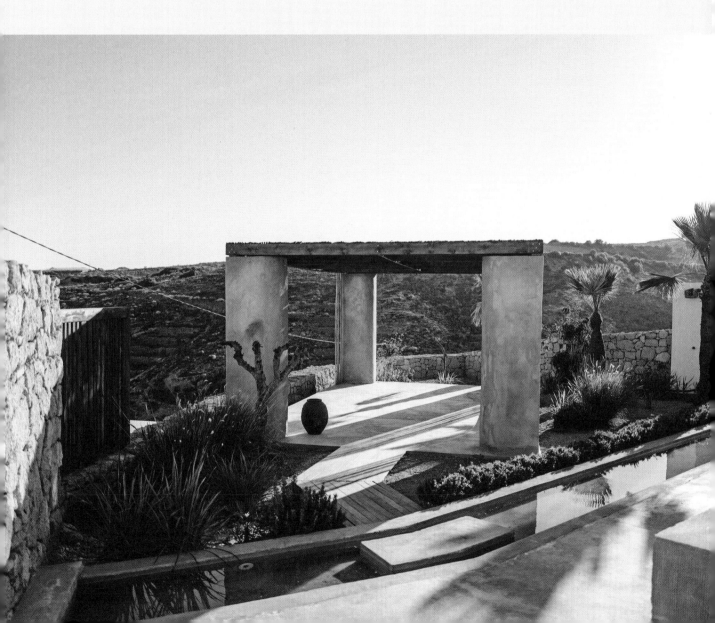

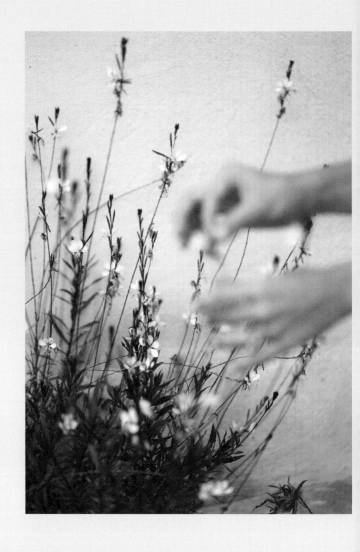

The hotel was once
crumbling farmland and
is now a sanctuary
for the body and soul.

In addition to this, the hotel offers a wide range of individual epigenetic therapies and naturopathy treatments led by a team of experts and centered on schools of homeopathy, phytotheraphy, aromatherapy, traditional Ayurvedic, as well as Chinese practices. Mealtimes at the hotel take place inside a mystic cave, where guests can choose from vegan, raw vegan, or vegetarian menus. Adhering to the farm-to-table philosophy, the chef is dedicated to sourcing the freshest, locally grown, and organic produce. Fresh seasonal fruits and vegetables, nuts, sea vegetables, and mushrooms regularly feature in the dishes he produces. For optimum nutrition and gut health these are supplemented with seeds and ferments such as sauerkraut, kefir, and sourdough bread.   *

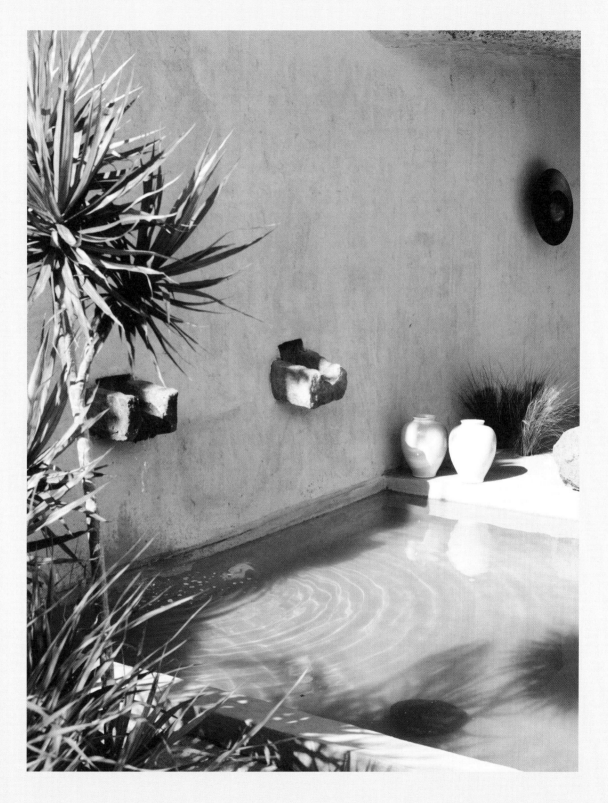

OPPOSITE AND ABOVE Owner Anthony Picq is an accomplished interior stylist and garden designer. His landscaping here is carefully considered and plants have been selected for their holistic properties. The lavender and rosemary is used at the retreat for making essential oils.

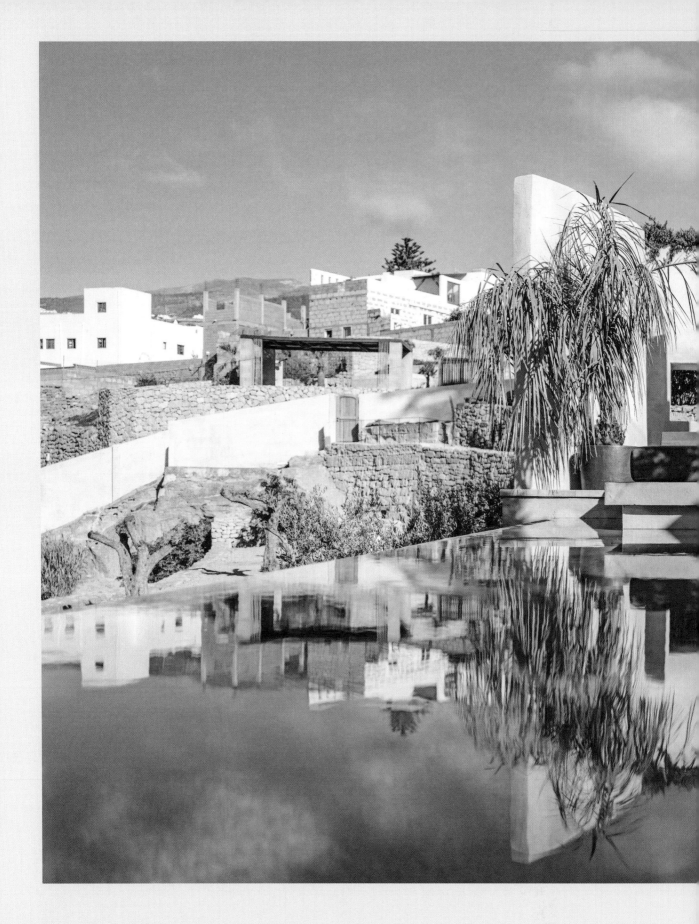

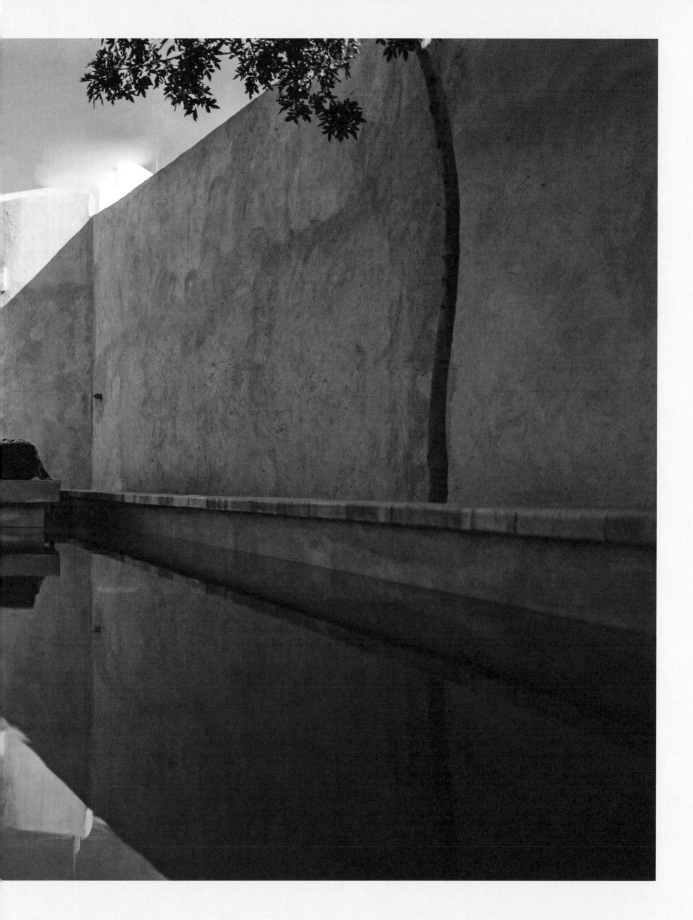

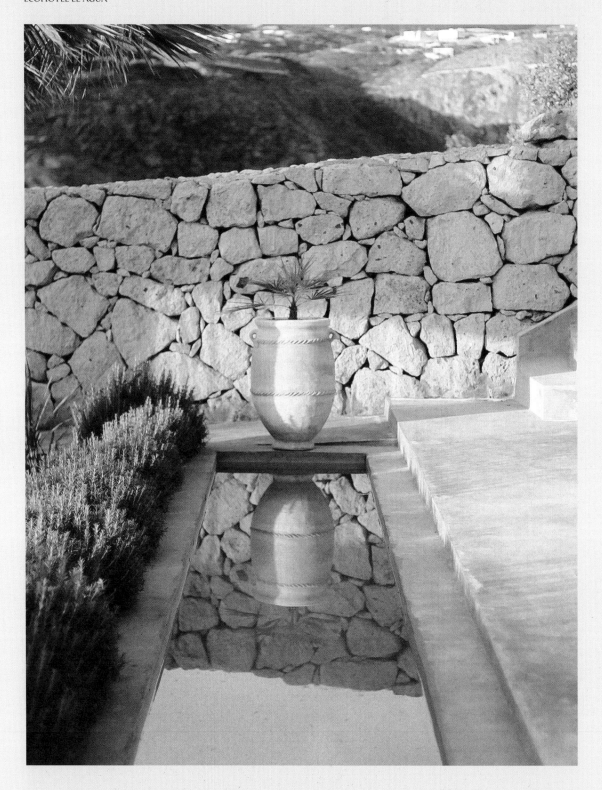

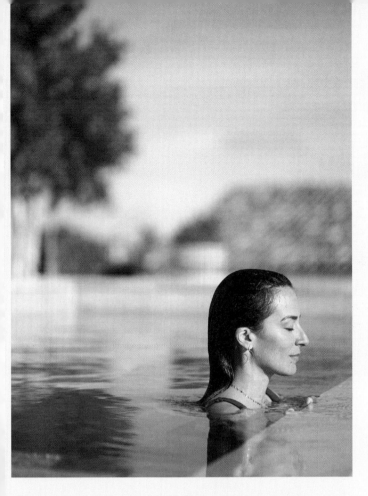

OPPOSITE AND LEFT Water features prominently throughout the resort. Whether the decorative channels that form part of the garden landscaping or therapeutic waters of the outdoor Jacuzzi and cold plunge pool, they inspire an opportunity for reflection as well as for healing.

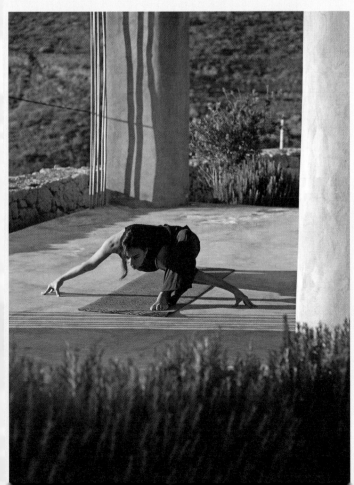

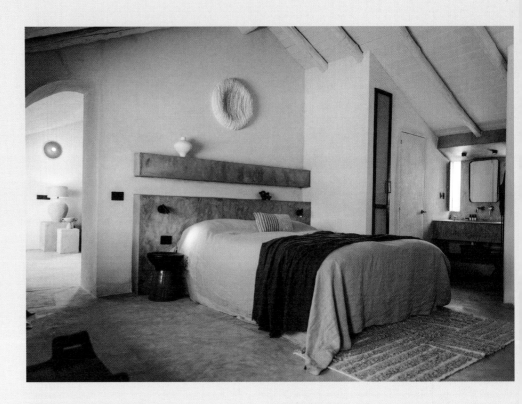

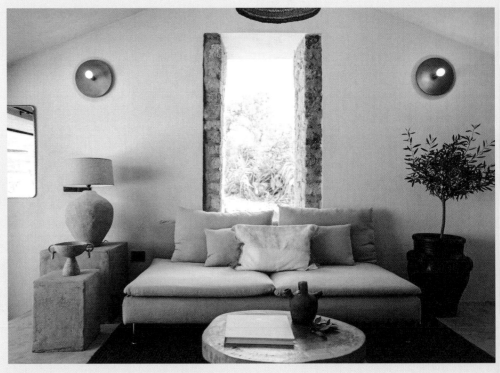

ABOVE AND OPPOSITE Guest accommodation has tastefully appointed interiors that pay homage to the surrounding landscape and tranquil outside spaces. Combining the principles of feng shui and *wabi-sabi*, they are rendered in a soft, neutral palette with natural textiles and furnishings.

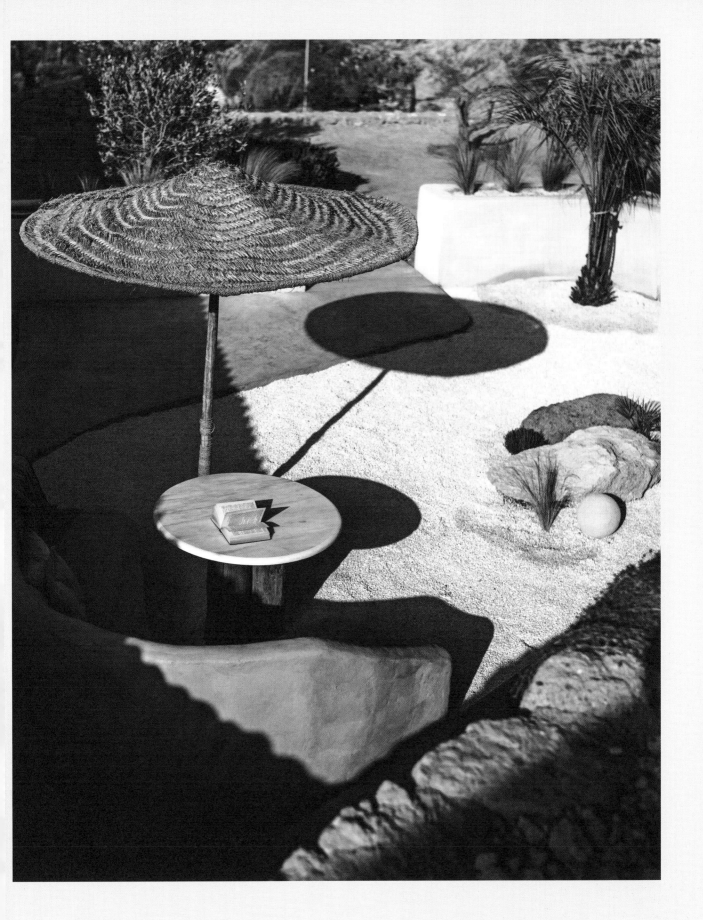

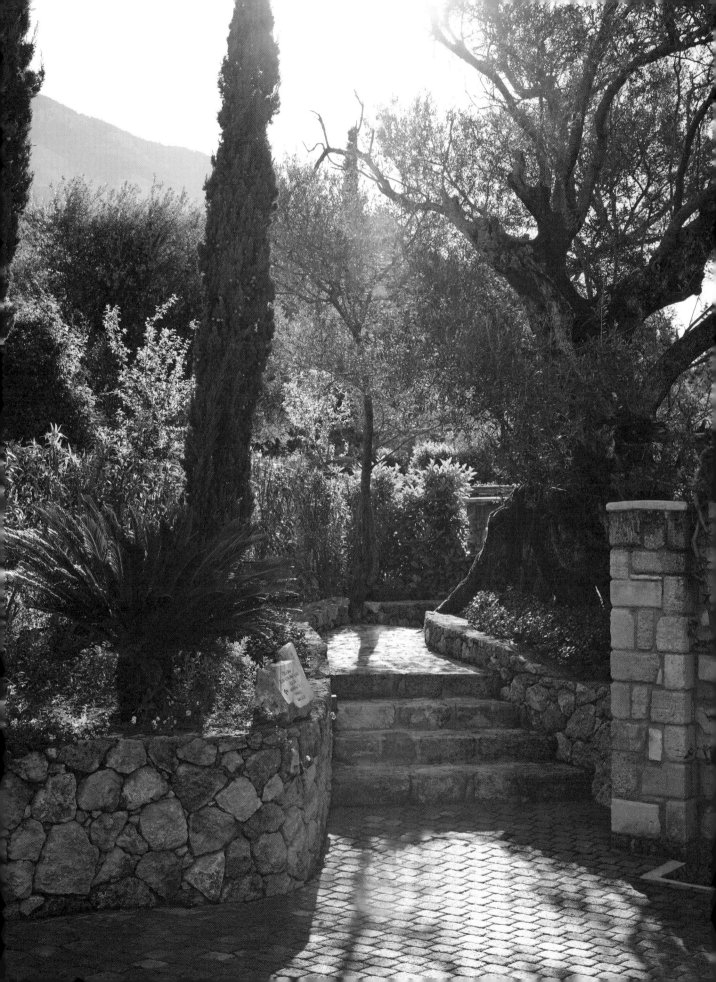

F Zeen Kefalonia

Livathos, Kefalonia, Greece

AN ISLAND IDYLL IN WHICH MIND, BODY, AND SOUL CAN TRULY ALIGN WITH NATURE

At this secluded Mediterranean resort, it does not take guests very long to FEEL AT PEACE *with themselves and the world around them and to appreciate the* SIMPLER THINGS *in life.*

According to the owners of this adults-only boutique hotel, "The good life starts here." They may have a point. Surrounded by lush vegetation on the Greek island of Kefalonia, and with access to unsullied beaches on the shores of the Ionian Sea, F Zeen is nothing short of paradise.

Striking a careful balance between luxury and simplicity, F Zeen accommodation is housed in a number of attractive properties nestled into the hilly island landscape, where the focus is on natural organic materials and hand-crafted finishes. Beautifully weathered stone walls, clay roof tiles, and timber decking are juxtaposed with hammered copper, marble finishes, and a neutral palette to create the most aesthetically pleasing of spaces. Blending in comfortably with their natural surroundings, almost all of the suites have immediate access to the outdoors—whether a private terrace, balcony, or garden—and several have their own pools or Jacuzzis. While some suites enjoy amazing panoramic views across the sea, others are a stone's throw from the beach, and one is immersed in the neighboring forest landscape. The names of the rooms give clues as to what to expect, among them Classic Garden Retreats, Terraced Penthouse Suites, and Superior Raw Retreats, and there is something for everyone.

While staying at the resort, guests can indulge in an impressive range of relaxing and rejuvenating treatments at the hotel's spa. Among the many items on the menu are a hammam steam bath, a Thai massage, and various seaweed-based wraps and scrubs, alongside a list of signature treatments that include sound healing therapy and a pure botanic detox. Guests also have access to

OPPOSITE Gardens were carefully designed to achieve a balance between the cultivated and the natural world. Enticing paths lead through spaces brimming with native vegetation.

three yoga decks—all in tranquil settings and within the sound of the sea. They can attend scheduled daily classes or book one-to-one sessions in meditation and vinyasa, hatha, and aerial yoga, among others. Additional physical activities aimed at increasing the well-being of hotel guests include outdoor fitness classes, tennis, hiking, snorkeling, and kayaking—all in the stunning and most serene of settings.

During their stay, guests are treated to mainly traditional Greek cuisine at the hotel's two restaurants, where there is an emphasis on fresh herbs and vegetables from on-site gardens. Menus feature fresh, organic ingredients prepared with care to nourish guests "from the inside out." The best time to visit this island resort is during the Mediterranean summer, from the month of May to October. ✳

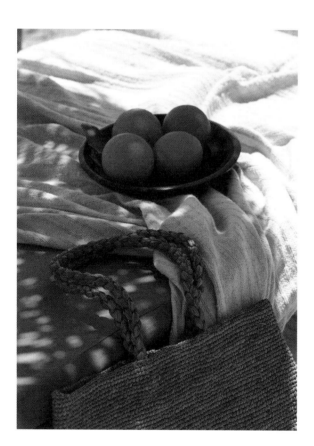
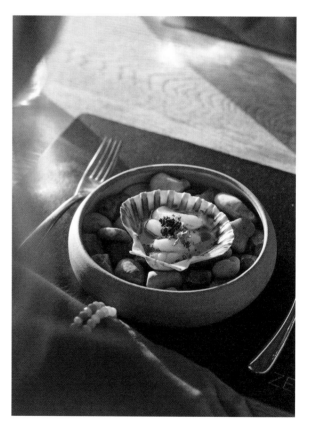

ABOVE Both of the on-site restaurants provide nourishing and balanced meals. Ingredients are locally sourced—many of them from the resort's own garden—and dishes are prepared using traditional techniques.

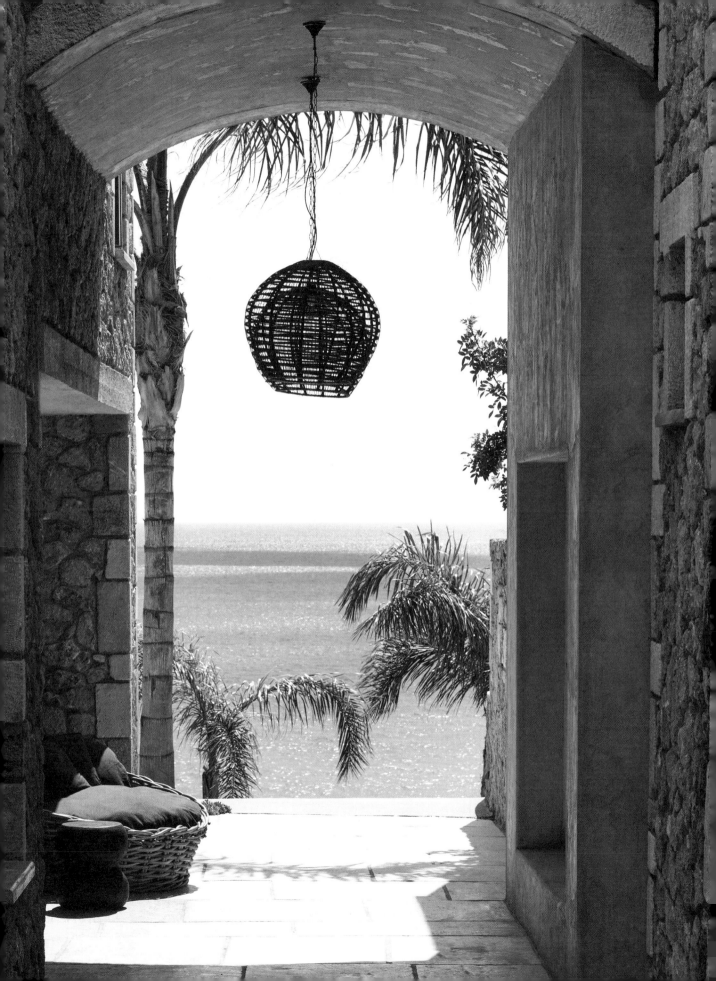

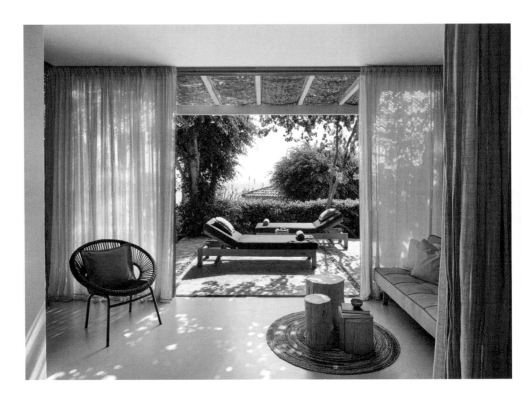

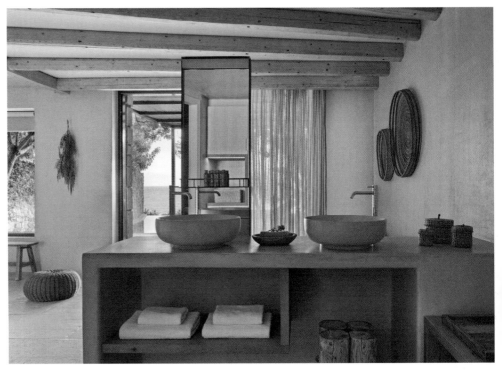

ABOVE Built to reflect the characteristics of the local architectural style, guest accommodation is predominantly made of stone and finished with natural materials. All rooms have sea and garden views and feel deeply immersed in the surrounding landscape.

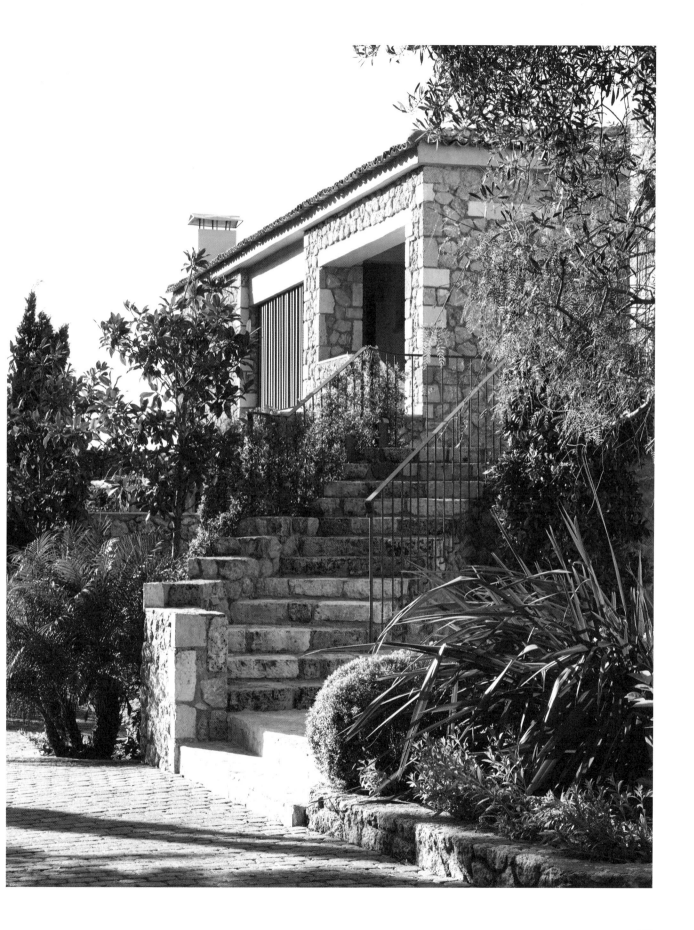

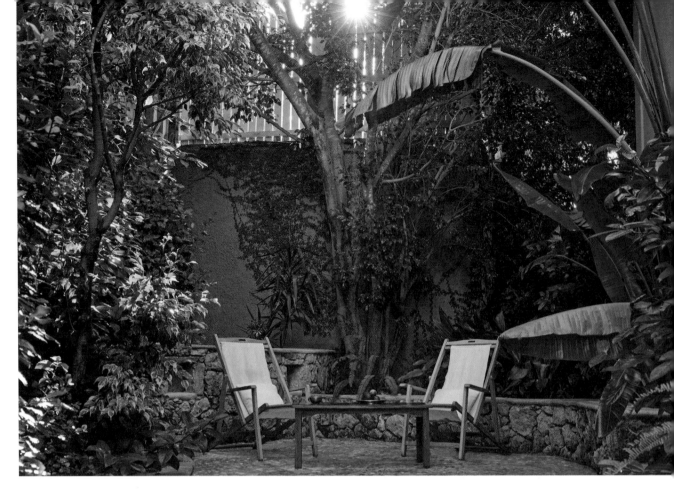

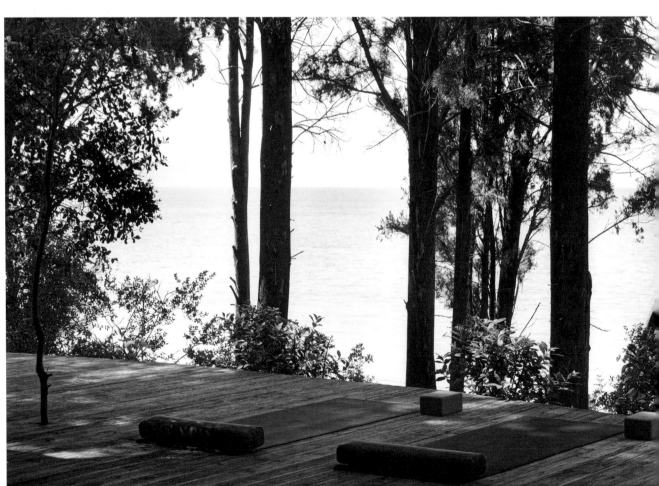

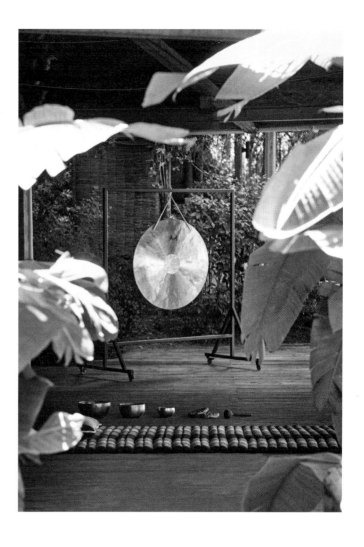

OPPOSITE AND ABOVE There is a great emphasis on being outside—yoga classes are held on one of four outdoor decks, and there is an outdoor gym with facilities for a wide range of activities from calisthenics to rowing. More tranquil spots across the grounds lend themselves to meditative therapies such as sound baths.

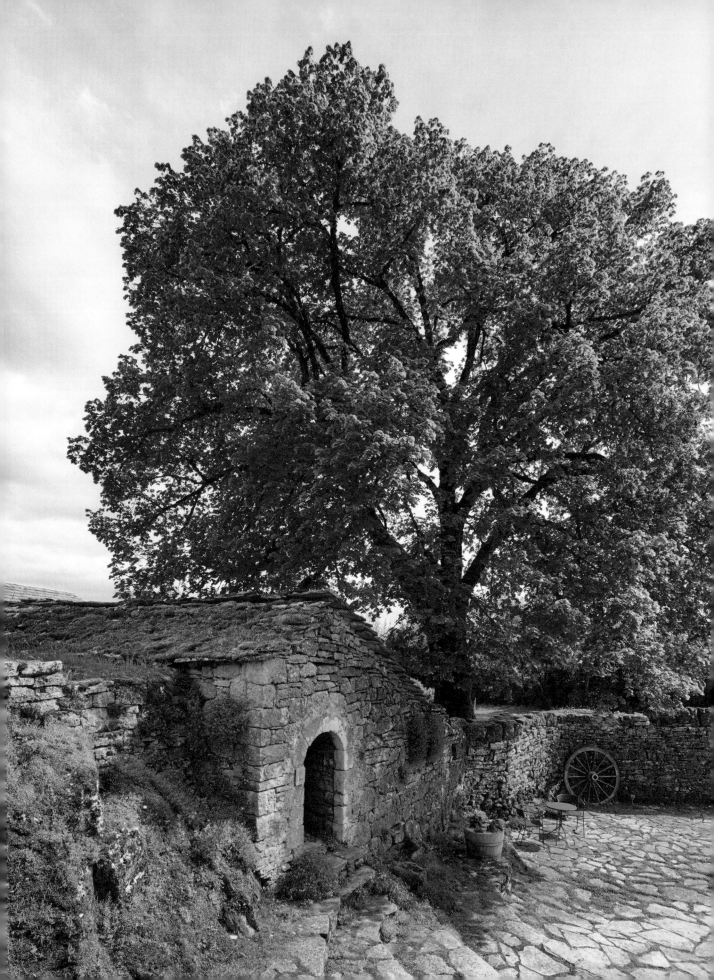

Almières
Lozère, France

TUNING IN TO THE SOUNDS OF NATURE IN A REMOTE AND RUGGED CORNER OF FRANCE

Set in a pretty 18TH-CENTURY HAMLET, Almières welcomes guests for five-day immersive retreats centered on yoga, meditation, and sound baths designed to help guests regain CLARITY OF MIND.

Perched on a cliff top in the Massegros Causses Gorges in southern France, the Almières retreat overlooks the dramatic Gorges du Tarn canyon, offering truly breathtaking views. The retreat is a collection of 18th-century stone houses on around 20 acres (8 hectares) of land, carefully restored by its owners. During the three-year renovation project, all choices of materials, suppliers, and partners were made to respect the property's history and environment, drawing on the expertise of local builders and craftspeople. This clutch of buildings feels like it has not changed for centuries, and there is an air of timelessness, a stillness, and a quietness broken only by the sounds of nature.

Set within a UNESCO World Heritage site, a designated Natura 2000 site, and a certified Dark Sky Reserve, the landscape around Almières is beautiful, rugged, and remote. There is no internet connection, making it the perfect spot for guests seeking to escape the modern world, to find time and space in which to relax and recharge—in the words of the retreat itself: "*to be* rather than to do." With accommodation for just 14 people, Almières offers five-day retreats with a focus on yoga and meditation. Guests have three options for rooms: the first, Casa Santiago, is a typical local house with stone walls and beautifully arched ceilings on the upper level. It has two bedrooms, overlooking the trees and gardens, a cozy living room with a wood-burning stove, and a shared bathroom. The second, the Lodge, is more spacious, with white-washed walls, beamed ceilings, timber floors, and plenty of room for two people. There are also four suites with private bathrooms. Here, too, the rooms have

OPPOSITE Faithfully restored by local craftsmen, the retreat buildings have changed little in appearance over the centuries. Their stone facades blend in beautifully with the surrounding landscape.

BELOW AND RIGHT Guest rooms are in newly built structures on the site, their design taking cues from the original buildings: stone floors and walls and rustic timbers. Modern technology allows for walls of glass, which add a contemporary twist.

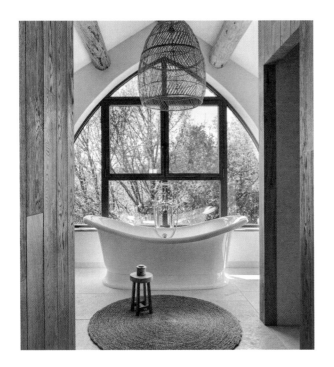

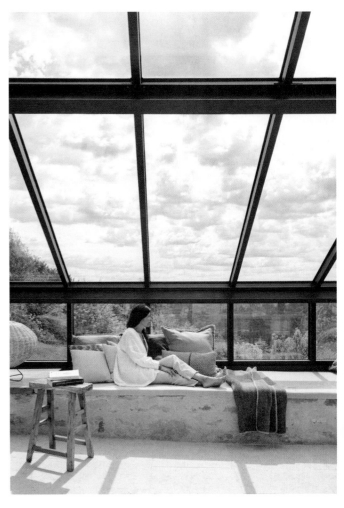

stone walls and arched ceilings. Much of the furniture and décor were sourced locally, and all textiles are natural.

Guests at Almières are invited to join a morning and evening yoga practice and a morning meditation session. An old stable has been converted into a treatment area where they can indulge in several health-benefitting treatments that include massages and saunas. There is an emphasis on the power of sound; sound massages and "meditative concerts" are offered to encourage a deep meditative state induced by the soft tones of Tibetan bowls, tuning forks, and gongs. All meals are inclusive, with menus centered on a plant-based cuisine. Retreats are themed according to the time of year, and are given romantic names that include New Breath of May, Autumn Nights, Swirling Leaves, and Just Before Winter. ✳

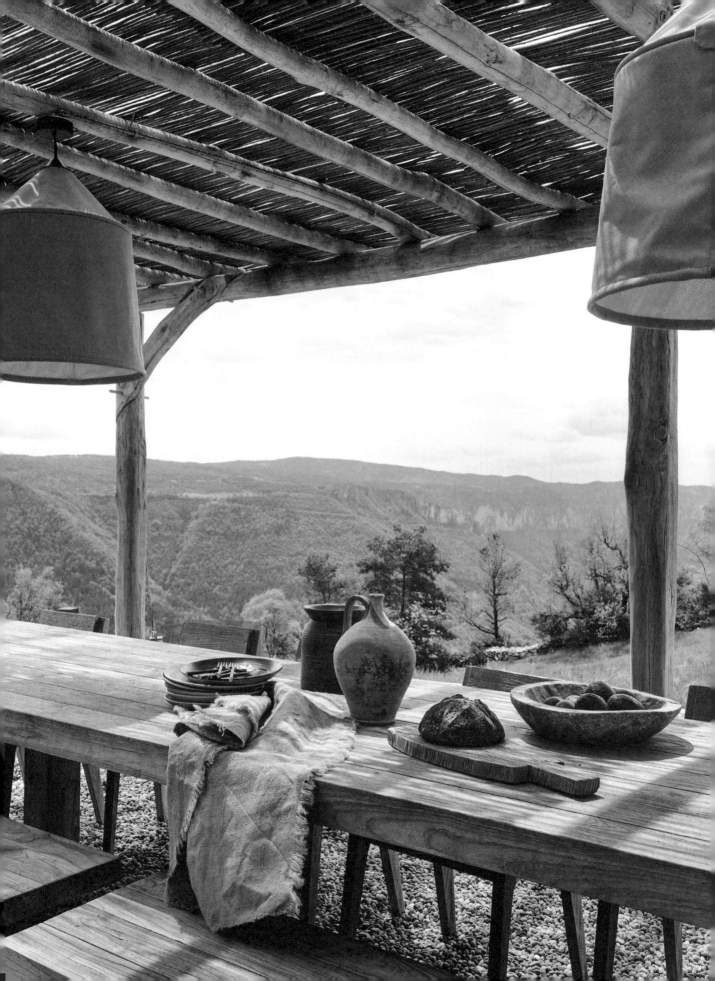

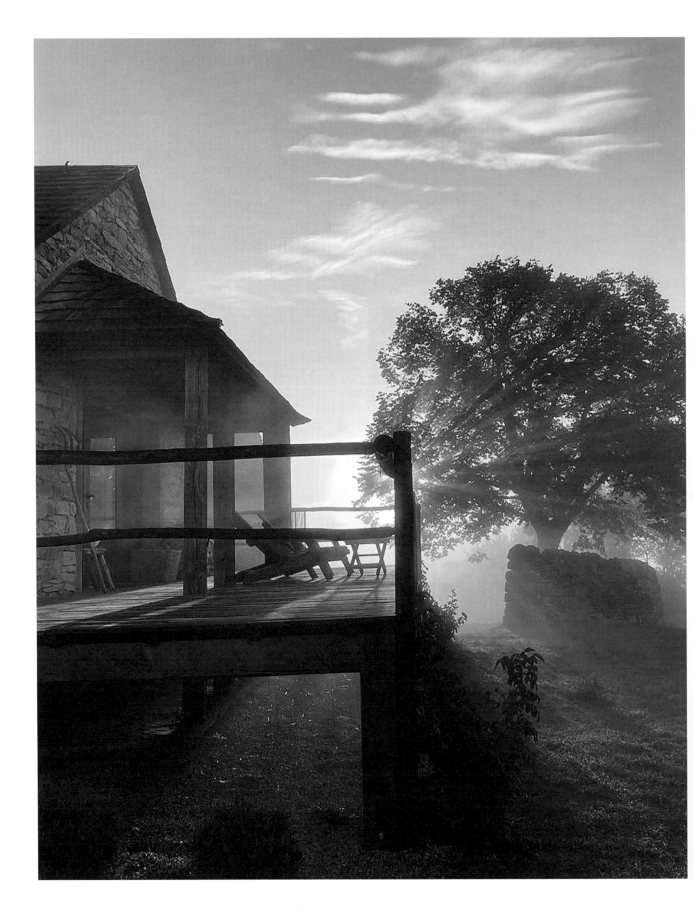

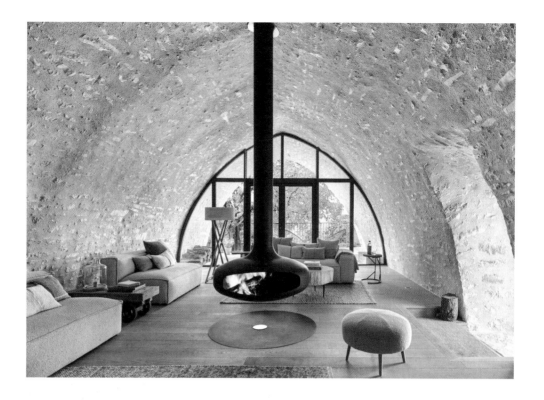

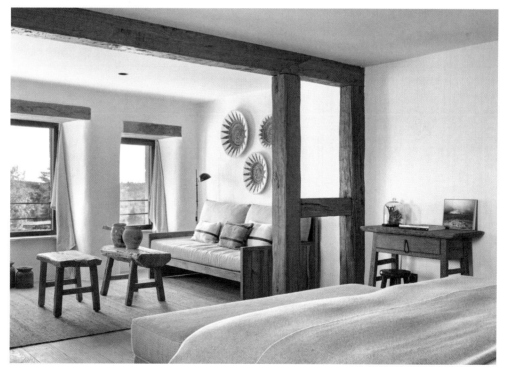

ABOVE Whether communal or private, all rooms across the complex are fitted out exquisitely and offer plenty of luxury to promote deep rest and relaxation. The décor achieves a comfortable blend of old and new in subtle, earthy tones.

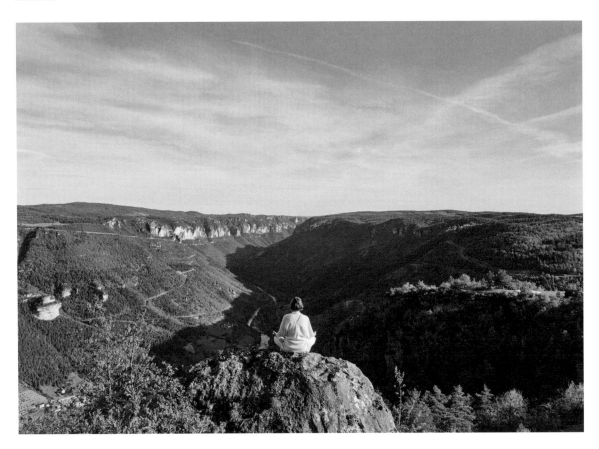

OPPOSITE The retreat is nestled in a dramatic landscape, and the owners have taken great care to preserve the character of the place. They landscaped the site in such a way that any new buildings, though reflecting the style of the old, are less visible on approach.

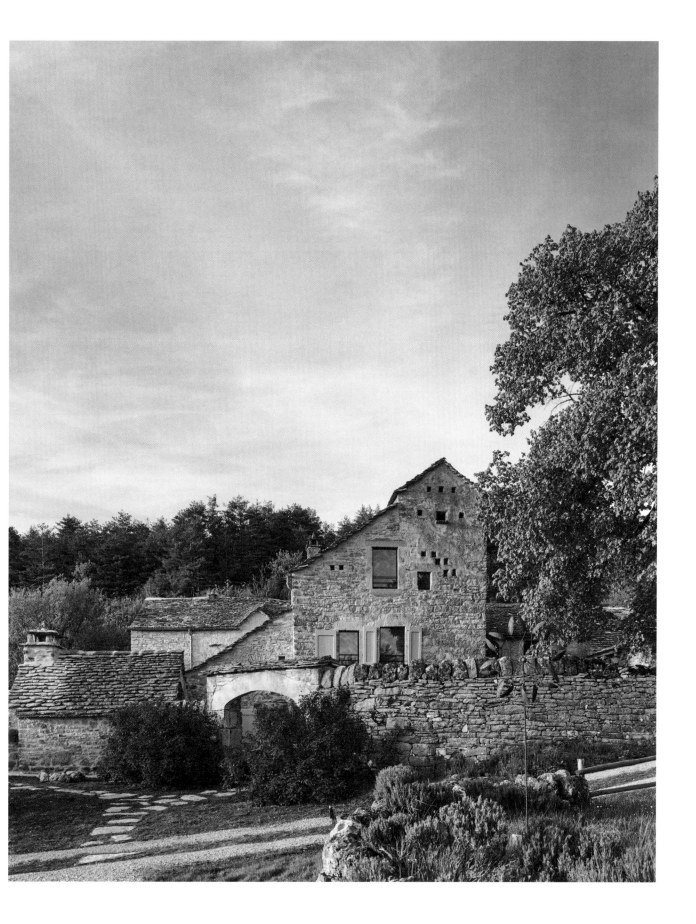

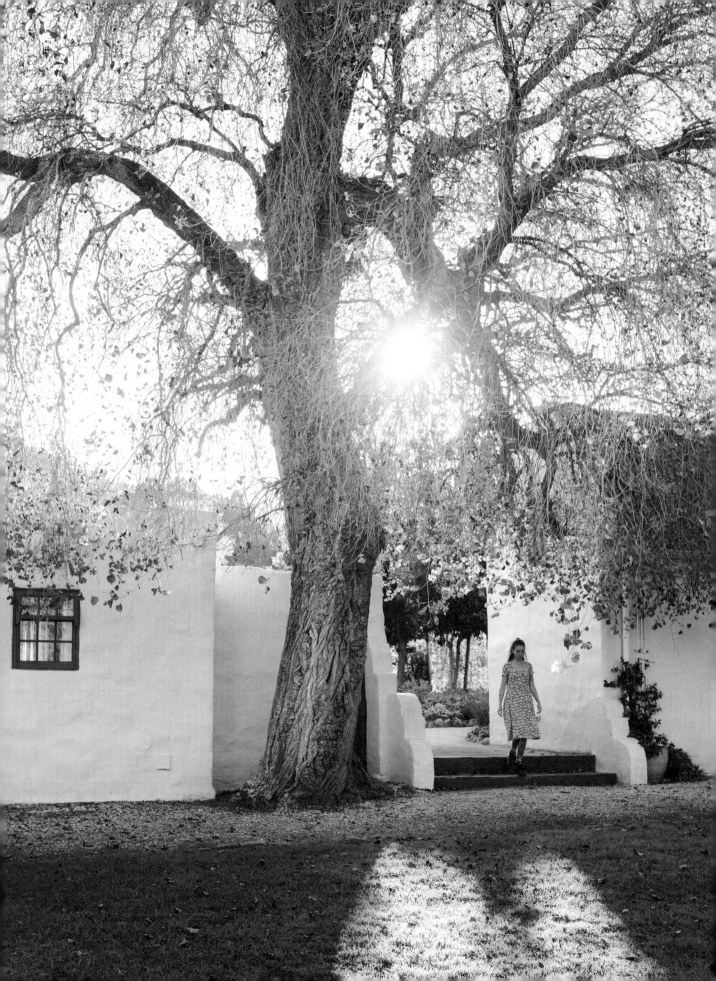

A WELL-BEING CENTER THAT FOSTERS CONNECTION TO THE SELF, OTHERS, AND NATURE

Bodhi Khaya Nature Retreat
Stanford, Western Cape, South Africa

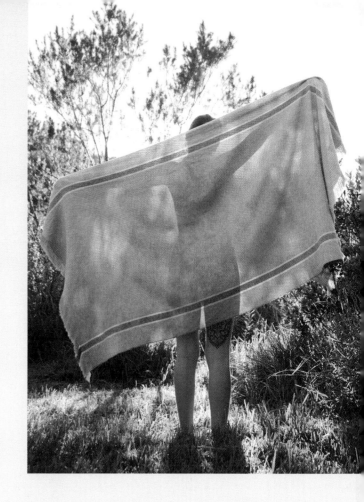

Nestled in the Overberg region toward the southernmost tip of the continent, daily yoga and meditation are the order of the day at this South African FARMLAND RETREAT surrounded by flora and fauna.

Around two hours southeast of Cape Town by road and at the foot of the Witkrans mountain, Bodhi Khaya Nature Retreat is in the heart of the Overberg region of South Africa. This is an area of great biodiversity and outstanding natural beauty, not far from the coast and characterized by rugged mountains and miles of *fynbos*—flora-rich shrubland. The retreat itself is situated on farmland and is a tranquil, rural spot in which to disconnect from the demands of city life and to reconnect with nature.

With a focus on meditation and contemplation, the resort offers a program of one-off retreats throughout the year in addition to its regular two- and three-night personal retreats available year-round. Offers include a three-day cleanse and detox, a three-day retreat led by a Buddhist monk that focuses on awareness, wisdom, and compassion, and a seven-day silent retreat. Guests booking in for a two- or three-night personal retreat can expect a daily schedule of meditation, yoga, and *chi kung* sessions. There are plenty of nearby trails for hiking and ponds for wild swimming, and the guests can take part in a tree-planting ceremony. All meals, which are plant-based, are included in the price, and the retreats offer massages, holistic coaching, private yoga, and breathwork as optional

OPPOSITE Across the estate, many of the buildings maintain the rustic charm of the original farmhouse and outbuildings, with simple whitewashed walls and green woodwork.

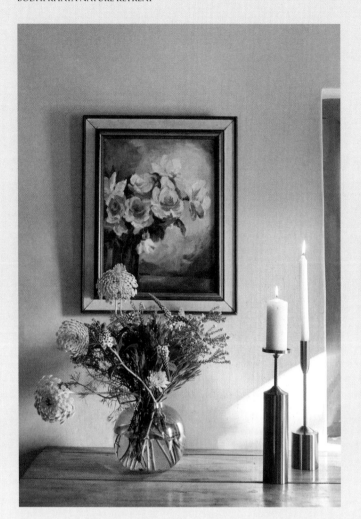

LEFT AND OPPOSITE Spaces inside and out are arranged for maximum comfort and relaxation. The colors used for decorating the rooms are rich, but also mellow, reflecting the hues found in the surrounding landscape. Dotted around the grounds are benches and hammocks.

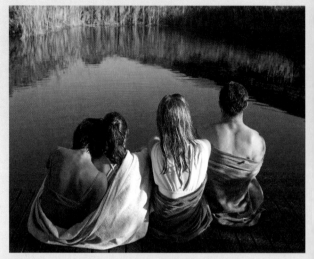

extras. Guests have a wide range of accommodation to choose from, the simplest being 14 monastery-style cloister rooms flanking a peaceful courtyard and furnished with little more than a single bed, a side table, and a small closet for clothing. Guests staying here have access to communal bathrooms and a generous open-plan living space that looks out across the gardens toward a labyrinth beyond. Close to the retreat's meditation hall, six courtyard rooms each sleep two and have en suite bathrooms. There are three rooms in the communal farmhouse and four garden rooms in the grounds. In a more remote corner of the farm and with views of the forest, the Wild Pod is a self-contained structure designed for hosting larger groups, with rooms for up to 10 people and a communal kitchen and lounge area. Finally, a short stroll from the retreat's main facilities and with access to a nearby swimming pool are two cottages that sleep four. All of the accommodation is beautifully decorated in the earthy tones of the surrounding countryside and many are

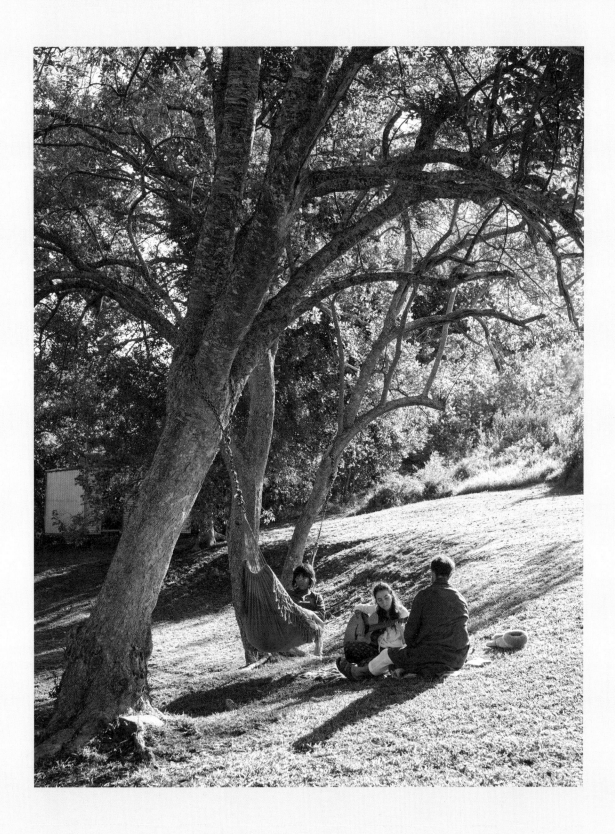

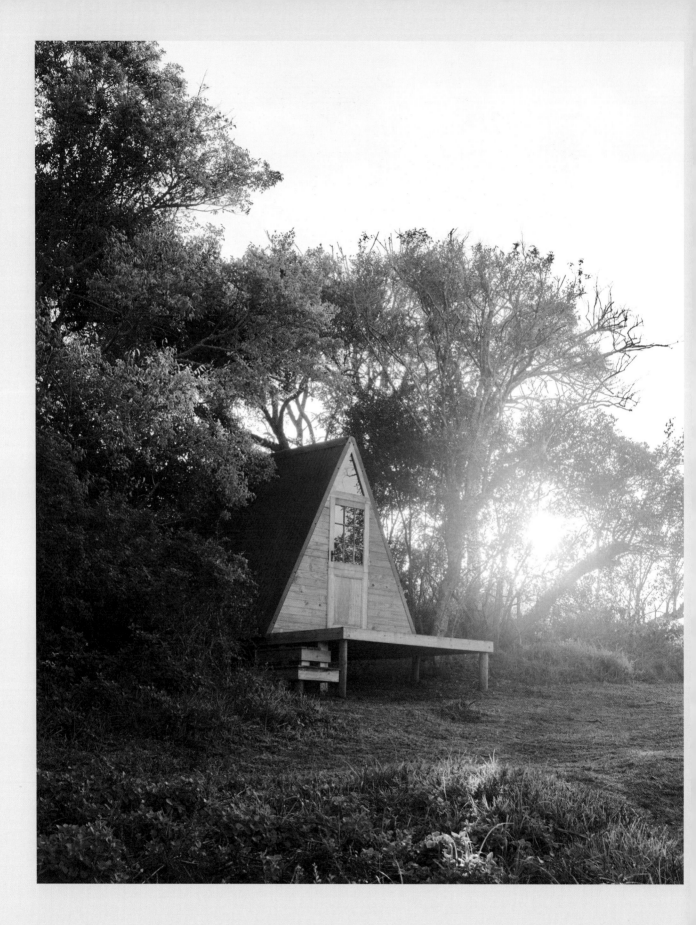

named for the local flora and fauna—Heron, Sunbird, Poppy, Fern, Wild Olive, Orchid, and Morning Glory.

This part of South Africa has a Mediterranean climate, which makes for a comfortable stay at any time of year. Besides the daily yoga and meditation sessions, winter sees guests gathering around cozy fireplaces after hiking one of the trails or taking a cold dip following a wood-fired sauna. Summer is for lazing on lush green lawns and swimming in a local spring-fed dam. Whatever time of year, there is always a calm and meditative atmosphere allowing anyone seeking peace and self-discovery to truly connect with nature. ✳

The accommodation
is beautifully decorated
in the earthy tones of the
surrounding countryside.

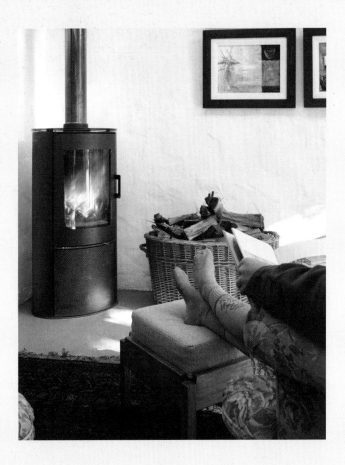

OPPOSITE The Wild Pod is set deep in the forest and has a communal kitchen and lounge area, plus a separate meditation hall with a yoga deck. Scattered around is a selection of A-frame cabins, caravans, and glamping tents that provide room for up to 18 people.

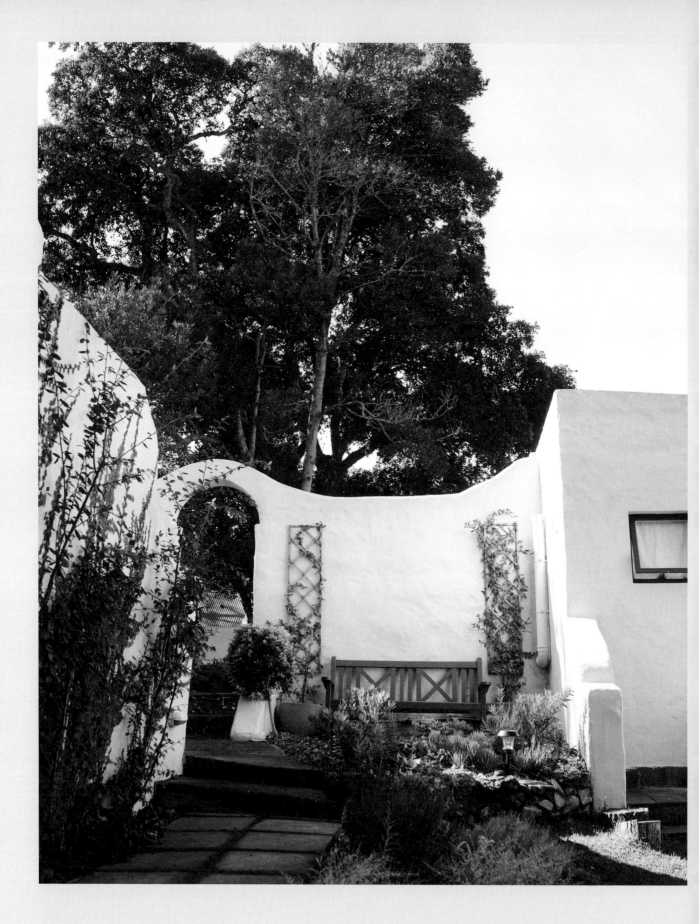

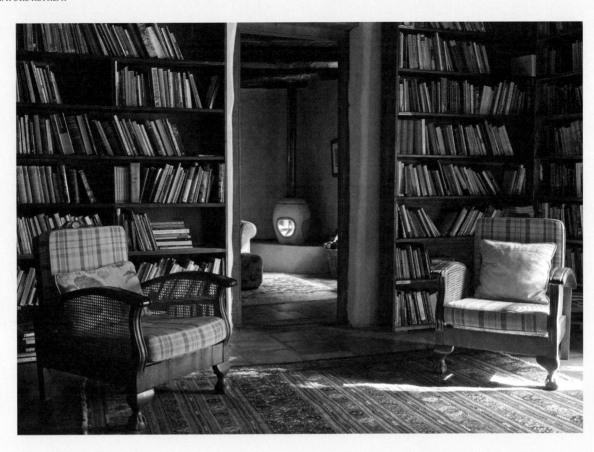

OPPOSITE AND ABOVE The main farmhouse has pretty communal spaces inside and out. Inside, they include
a kitchenette, a cozy lounge with a fireplace, and a charming, well-stocked library with armchairs for whiling
away an hour or two with a good book.

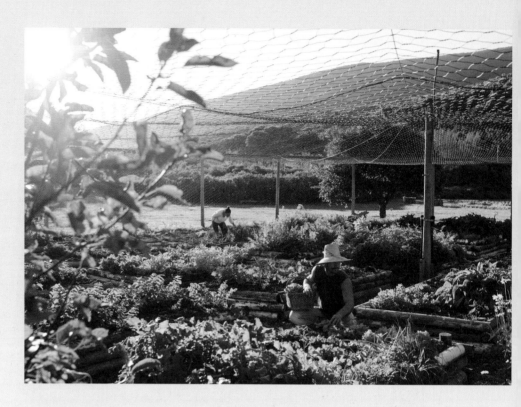

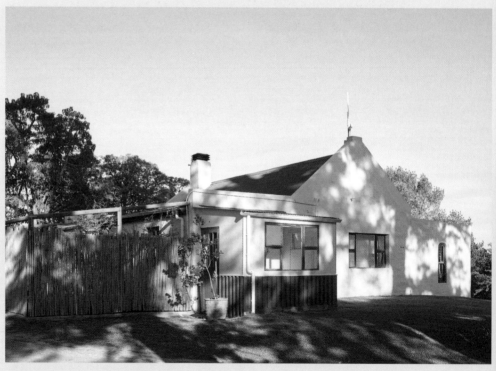

TOP The retreat has extensive gardens in which much of the kitchen produce is grown. ABOVE Sunbird Cottage is a short stroll from the retreat center and offers self-catering accommodation for up to four guests. OPPOSITE The complex that houses the four Garden Rooms.

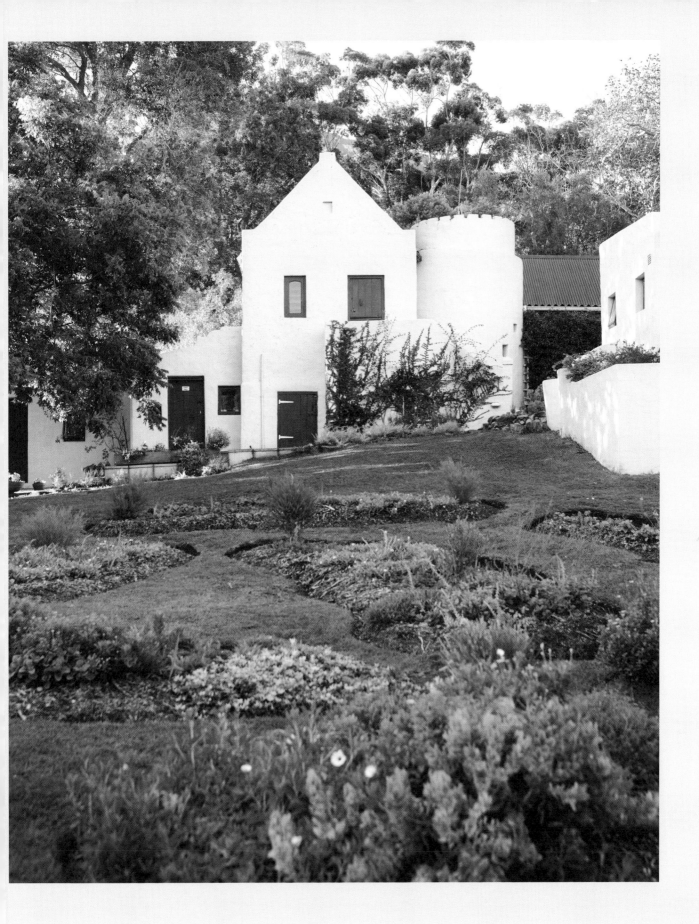

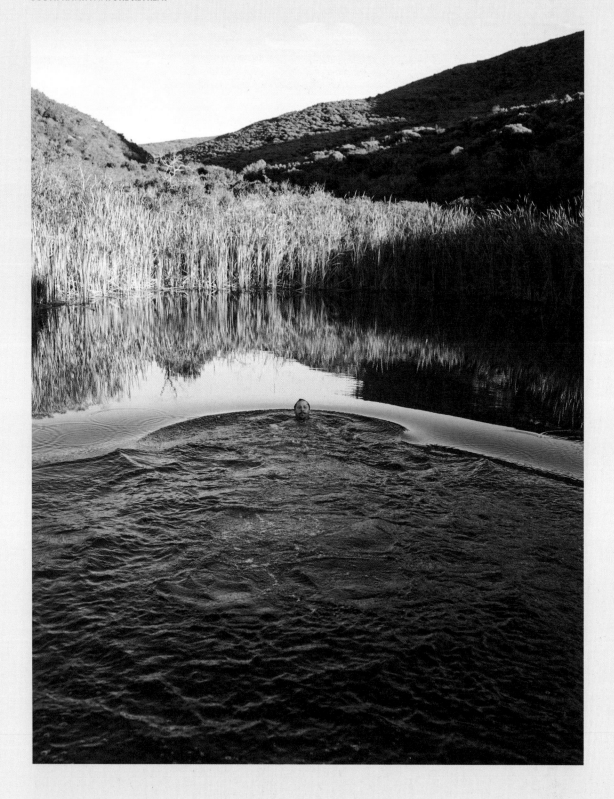

The retreat is situated on
farmland and is a tranquil,
rural spot in which to
reconnect with nature.

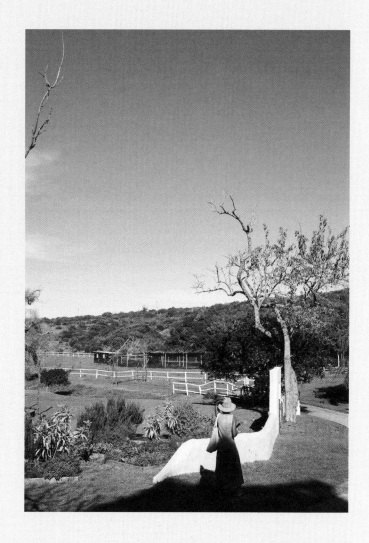

OPPOSITE AND ABOVE The retreat is in the Walker Bay Fynbos Conservancy, an area of incredibly rich biodiversity. The owners
have made a conscious effort to maintain a balance between areas of wilderness and the landscaping around the farm buildings.

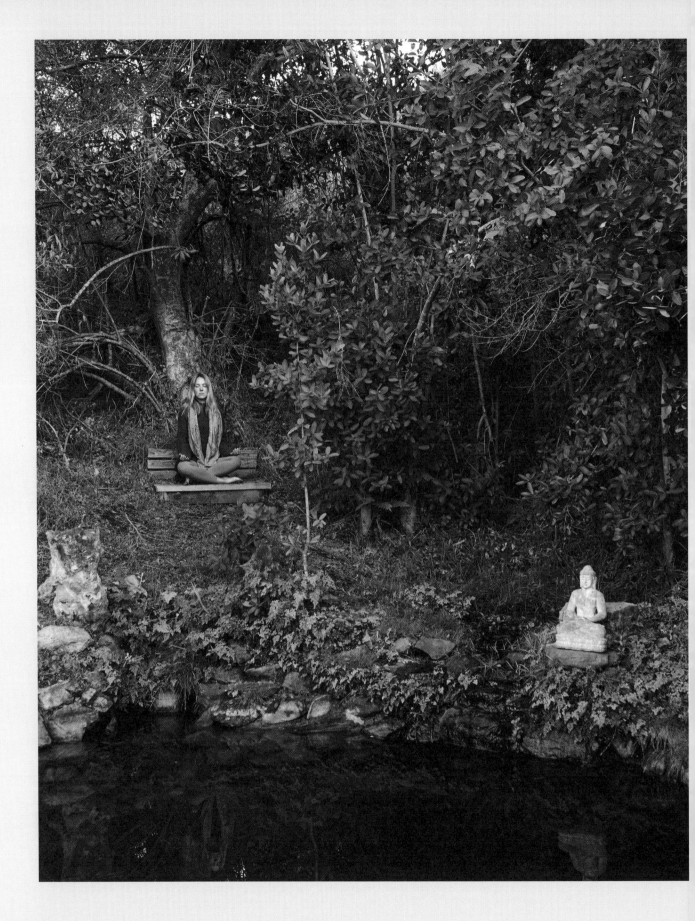

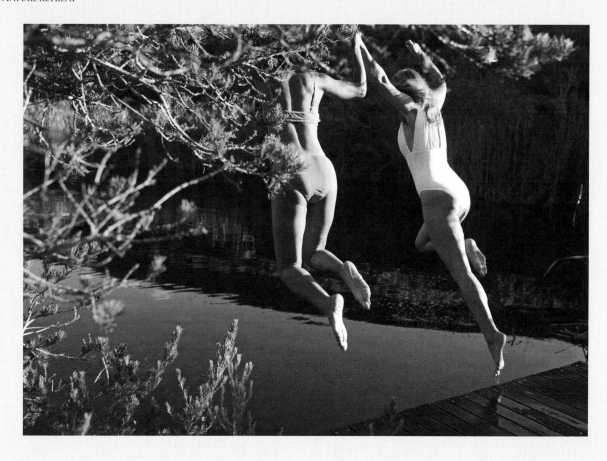

OPPOSITE AND ABOVE During the two- and three-night stays, guests enjoy a daily schedule of soul-nourishing meals, meditation, yoga, and *chi kung* classes. They are also encouraged to spend time walking in nature, swimming, and resting under the shade of a tree.

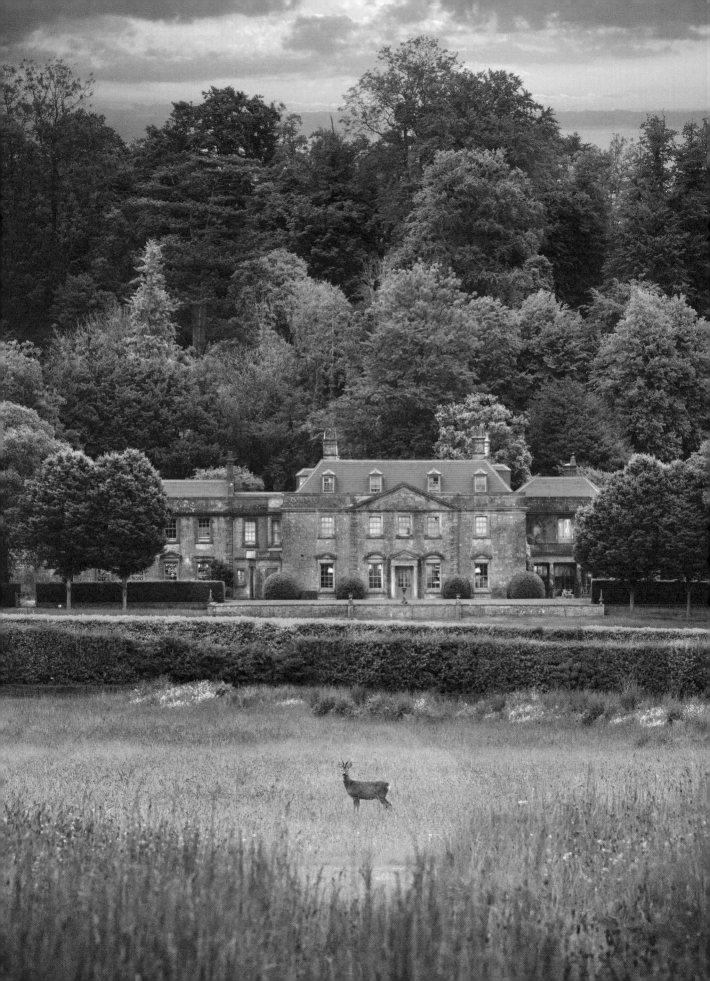

LUXURIOUS SPA TREATMENTS IN THE MOST BUCOLIC OF SURROUNDINGS

The Newt in Somerset
Bruton, U.K.

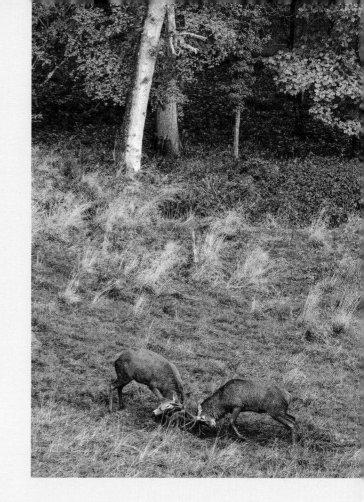

At this award-winning BOUTIQUE HOTEL, *guests can wind down on sun terraces, take high tea in the library, fine-dine in one of three restaurants, and indulge in a wide range of* RELAXING SPA TREATMENTS.

The Newt in Somerset is a luxurious boutique hotel on a working 1,000-acre (400-hectare) estate that features immaculate, carefully tended gardens, orchards, rolling valleys, and wild woodland. At its heart is Hadspen House, a handsome Georgian manor house which, together with its Stable Yard, accommodates 23 comfortable guest rooms. An additional 17 guest rooms are located in the Farmyard, in buildings that once served as a threshing barn, a cheese barn, a stable, a granary, and a cider press—all sensitively converted and retaining many of their original features. Throughout the estate, no two rooms are the same. Some have stone walls,

others have loft-style rafters, some have king-size four-poster beds, others have rolltop bathtubs. They are all beautifully decorated and have en suite bathrooms and stunning views out across the estate and beyond.

The estate has not one but three exceptional restaurants, all centered on farm-to-table dining with much of the produce grown or foraged on the estate. At the top end, the Botanical Rooms in the main Hadspen House offers elegant seasonal dining inspired by, and sourced from, the local area. The Farmyard Kitchen, housed in the old threshing barn, serves hearty, comforting dishes meant for sharing. The Garden Café

OPPOSITE At the heart of the estate, Hadspen House was built in the 17th century and remodeled during the 18th century. Today, it retains the essence of a Georgian family home.

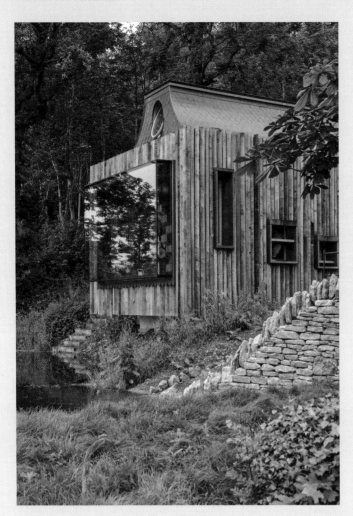

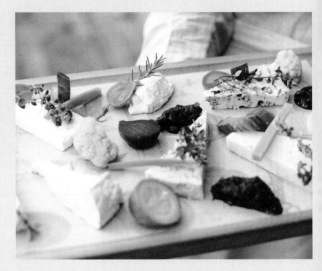

LEFT The Beezantium is a striking lakeside apiary for honey bees. Housing several hives that were built into its walls, the structure also serves as an exhibition space for hotel guests and visitors to the gardens. BELOW The Cured Matured Board, from the Garden Café menu.

overlooking the kitchen gardens and orchards offers lighter meals, which include breakfast and cream teas.

Between mealtimes, guests can indulge in a wide range of health-promoting classes and treatments at the hotel spa. These include yoga sessions, breath workshops, and sound healing; bespoke herbal body-cleansing and facial therapies inspired by the Newt's own Medicinal Herb Garden; deeply relaxing massages; and use of a hydro pool, steam room, and sauna. Particularly noteworthy are the spa's hammam treatments, held in a private marble-lined room, and inspired by both the Moroccan and Turkish traditions. The deeply cleansing treatments use natural products such as honey and milk to leave guests feeling revitalized, nourished, and relaxed. The Newt spa welcomes day trippers, but a two-night stay allows guests to benefit fully from all this award-winning boutique hotel has to offer.

In recent years, the estate owners have crafted a Four Seasons Garden not far from the Farmyard. Arranged as four distinct plots, the garden reflects the best of each season's

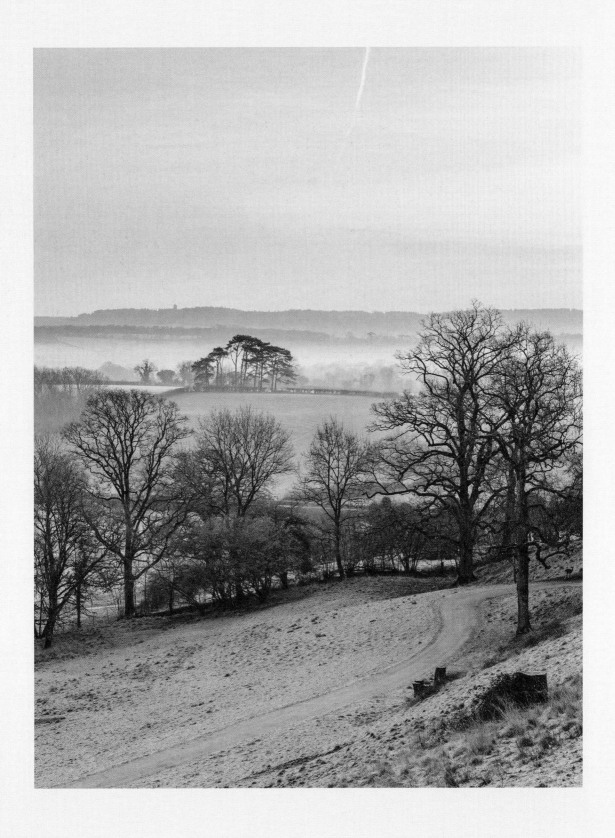

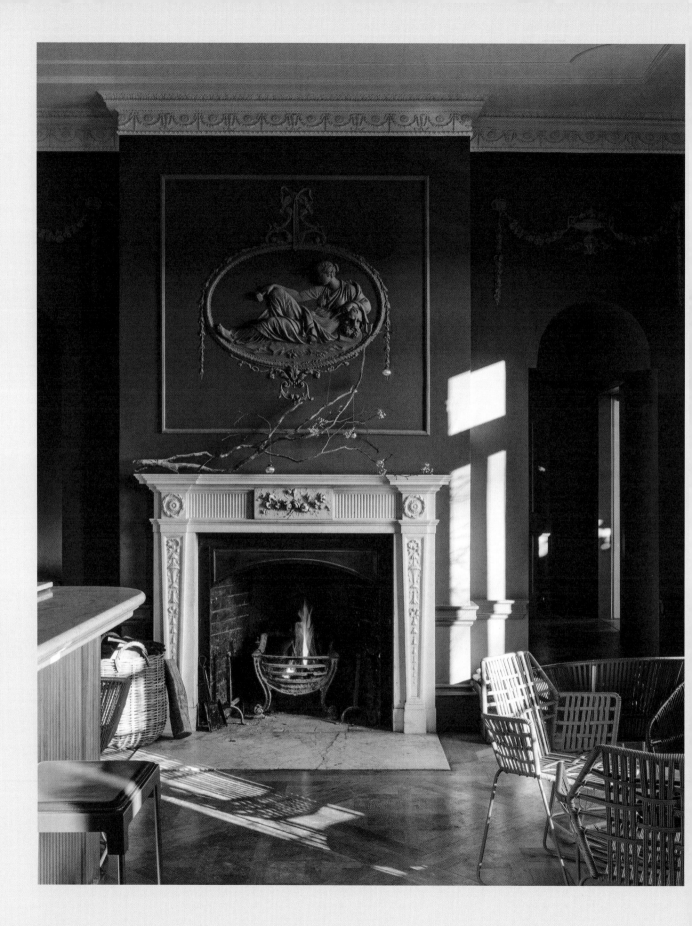

At the heart of the hotel is Hadspen House, a handsome Georgian manor house.

flora so that whatever the time of year, there are plants that are reaching the peak of their beauty. The summer garden, for example, features lavender hedges and roses in soft, romantic hues that wind around pergolas and climb walls. At the garden's center is a full-size cast of the Peter Pan statue that stands in London's Kensington Gardens. Accessed via a scenic path that passes through the kitchen gardens and apple orchards, this experience alone is enough to make guests feel at one with nature and totally relaxed within their surroundings. ✳

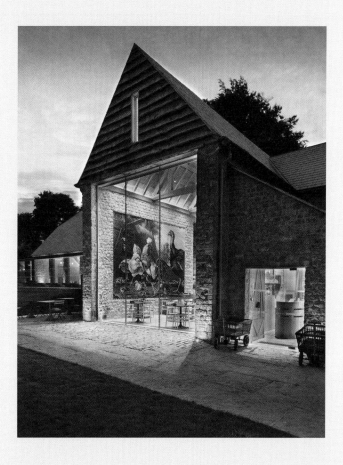

OPPOSITE The bar in Hadspen House has a stately feel to it, with its dark green décor and open fire, although the contemporary bar and furnishings add a lighter touch. ABOVE The Farmyard Kitchen, with its impressive floor-to-ceiling windows.

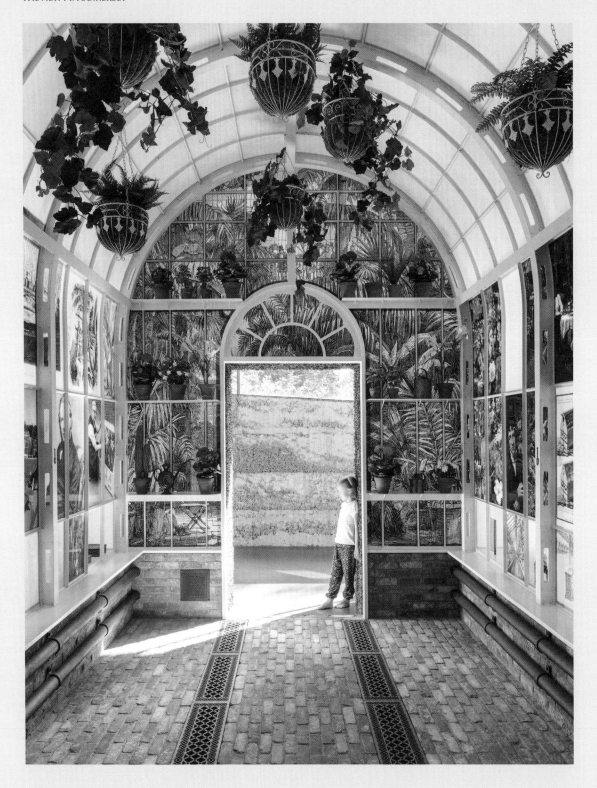

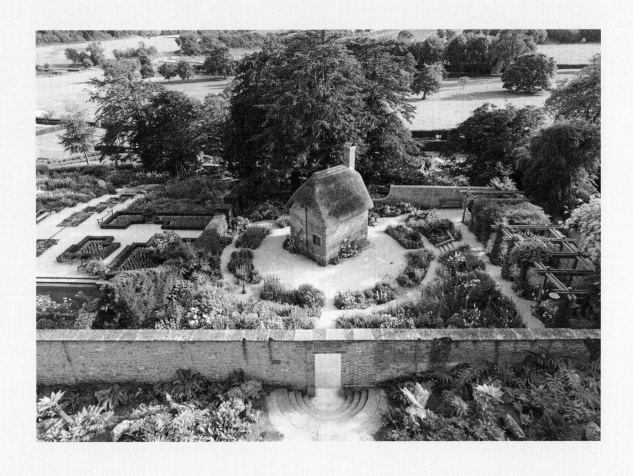

OPPOSITE The Story of Gardening exhibition space offers guests a history of gardening through interactive displays.
ABOVE Cottage-garden-style planting surrounds a restored, thatched gardener's cottage in the estate's Kitchen Garden.

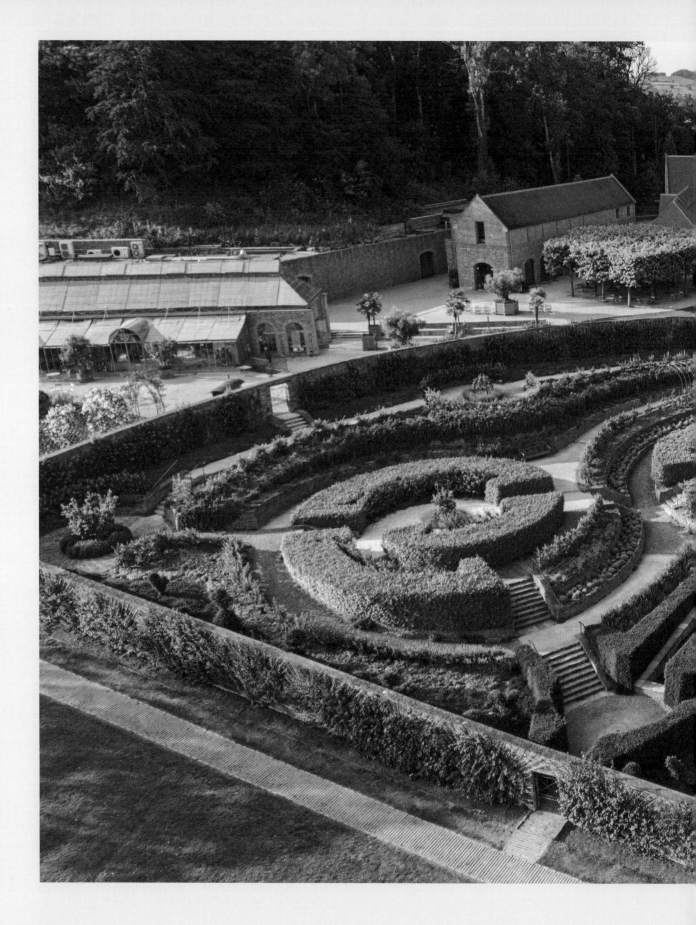

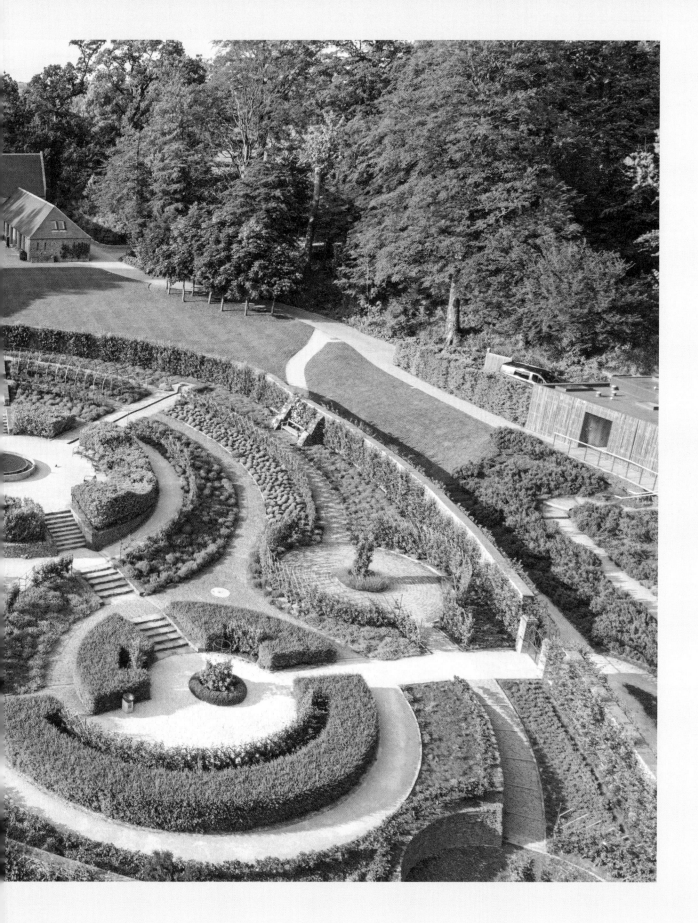

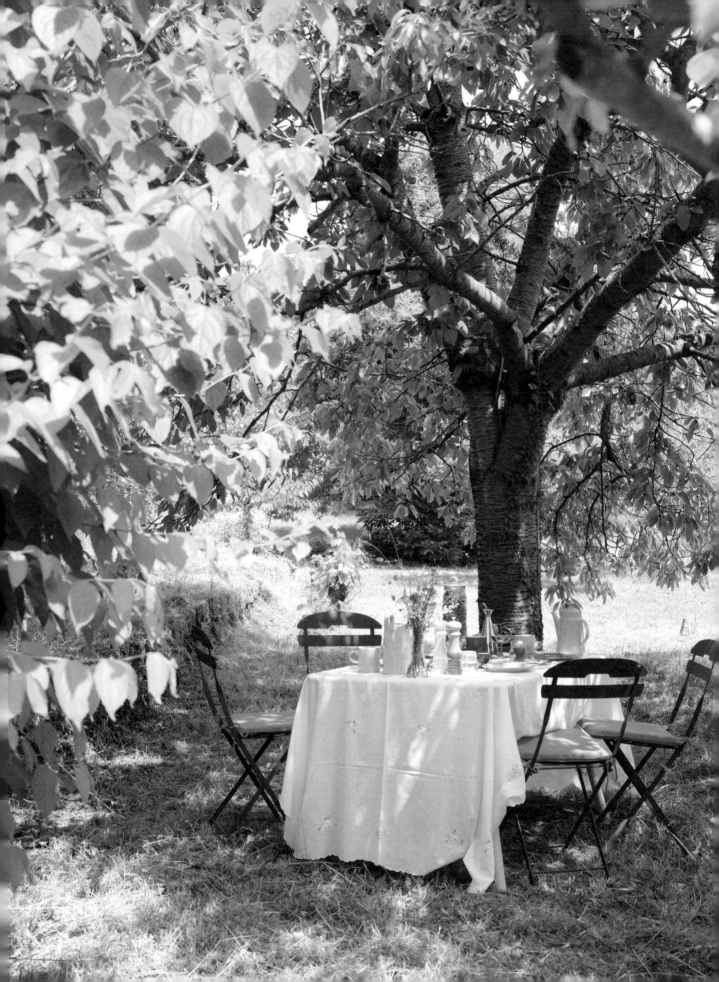

Casa Lawa
Catania, Sicily, Italy

A WHOLESOME FOODIE PARADISE ON THE SLOPES OF MOUNT ETNA

During a four-day CULINARY RETREAT led by the chef-in-residence, guests combine taking trips to the local market with making new friends, learning new skills, and RELAXING in the Sicilian sunshine.

The rural idyll of Casa Lawa is a small collection of early 19th-century single-story stone buildings sitting on 25 acres (10 hectares) of land in the foothills of Mount Etna, Sicily. The estate was once a vineyard and the terraces are still there, though now they are planted with fruit trees. Etna might be the world's most active stratovolcano, but this spot, almost 3,000 ft (900 m) above sea level, is perfectly tranquil. There are views across to Mount Etna on one side and out toward the sea on the other, and the coast is just 25 minutes away.

Polish-born Lukas Lewandowski, a former stylist, gallerist, and chef who worked in Berlin and Amsterdam, opened Lawa as a space where he could combine his love of cooking with his passion for design and hospitality. The guesthouse, itself built from volcanic rock, originally housed a grape press and is now home to four suites, named either Sea Room or Volcano Room according to the view that greets guests from their windows. Italian furnishings alongside colorful midcentury and postmodern pieces adorn the suites with their terracotta or timber floors and high beamed ceilings. Both types of rooms have a private bathroom, and the more spacious Volcano Rooms also have their own private entrance and a separate living room area.

A stay at Casa Lawa revolves around food. Central to the operation is a residency program where a rota of international chefs changes throughout the year. Residencies have included Hannah Kleeberg from Herrlich Dining in Berlin and Australian pastry chef Elisabeth Wynne. According to the owners: "As people from different

OPPOSITE In the summer months, guests start their day with a wholesome breakfast simply laid out on a table in the cherry orchard.

countries and heritages, they approach the soil, the ingredients, and the Italian culture through new eyes." The chefs have at their disposal a 4-acre (1.6-hectare) kitchen garden and an orchard with some 300 cherry trees. Menus typically focus on fresh local produce and predominantly plant- and fish-based dishes.

With just eight guests staying at a time, a vacation here is intimate and convivial, with people gathering around the table three times a day. Here they share stories of their daytime activities, whether driving to the sea for a swim, hiking the local terrain, or, in winter, taking to the ski slopes.

In recent years, Casa Lawa has organized a number of dedicated four-day retreats that focus on baking and fermenting. Guests also have the opportunity to take part in food-related excursions such as dining on the beach, visiting a provolone dairy, and joining a wine-tasting class.　✳

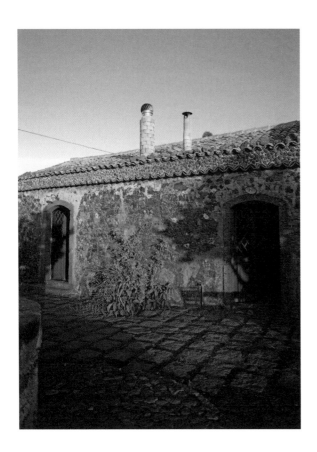

ABOVE Guests often share meals on the terrace outside the lava-stone guesthouse. OPPOSITE The volcano rooms have their own private living rooms—cozy spaces with beamed ceilings, stone floors, and an eclectic mix of rustic and midcentury furnishings.

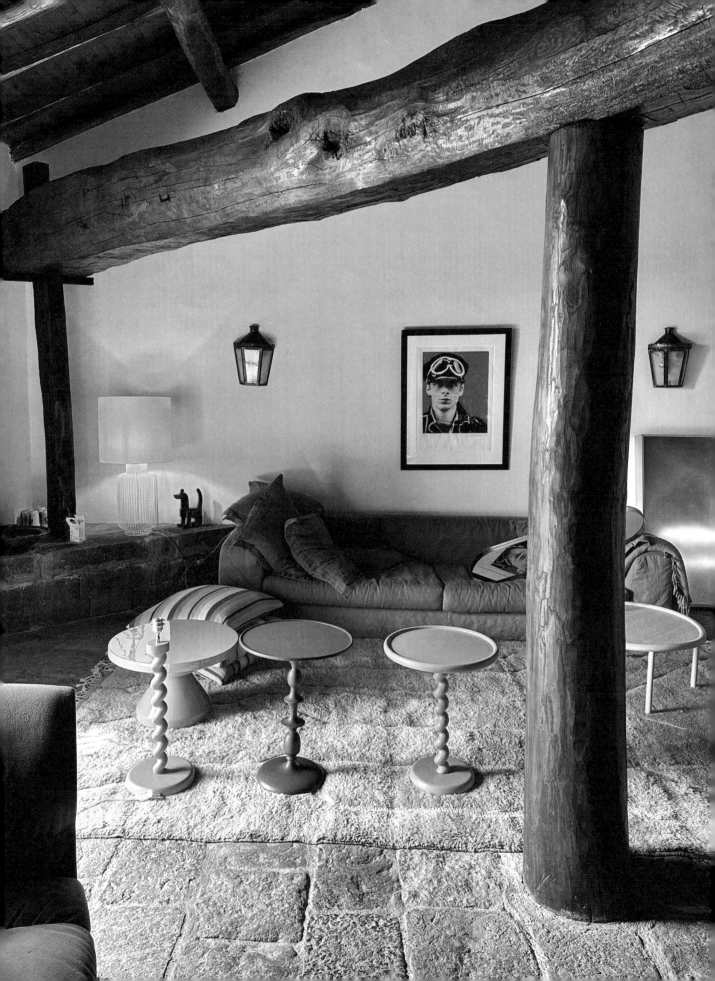

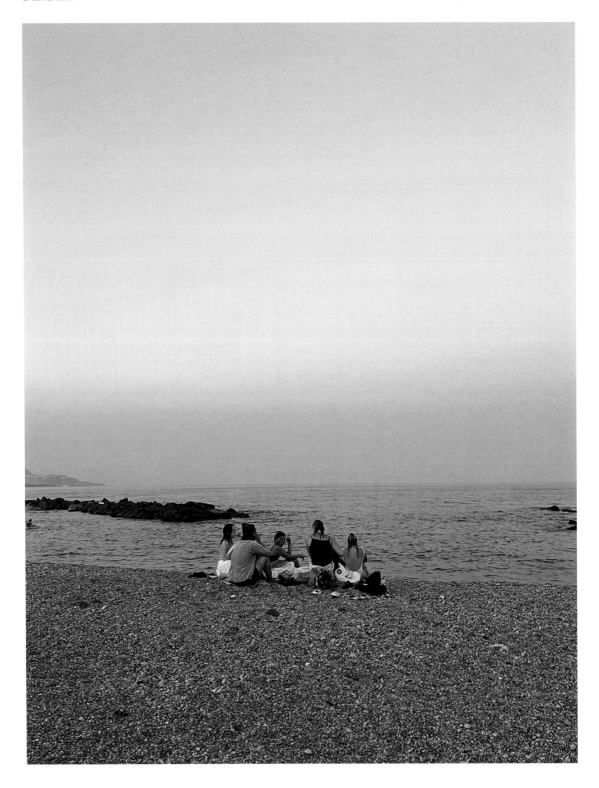

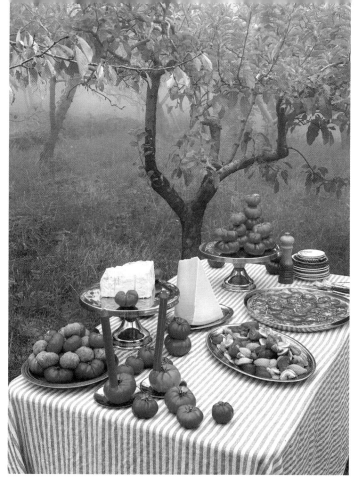

OPPOSITE Guests can spend time at the beach, which is just 25 minutes away from Casa Lawa. LEFT AND BOTTOM Part of the fun at this retreat is the ever-changing rota of guest chefs through the year, as each has their own take on how to use the locally sourced produce.

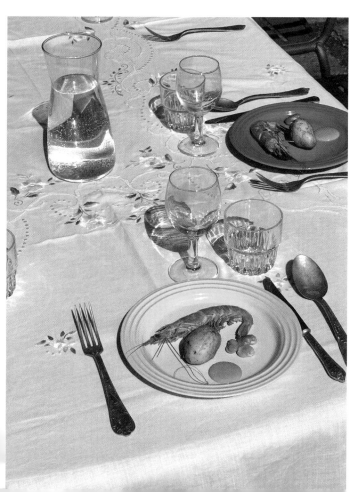

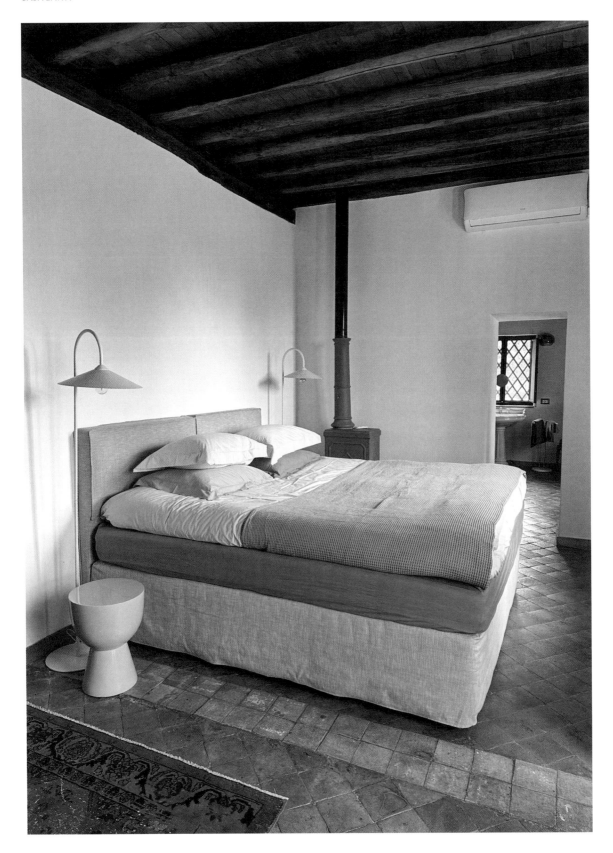

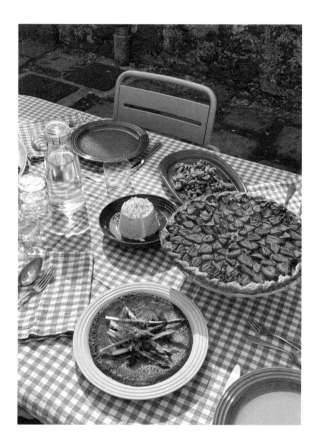

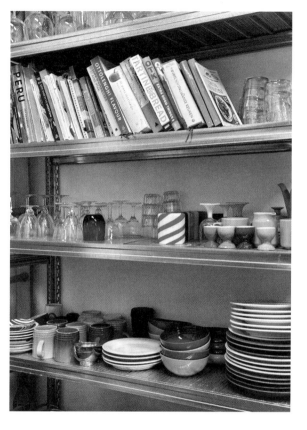

OPPOSITE AND ABOVE This retreat is all about color. From the ceramic tableware on the kitchen shelves to the linen in the bedrooms, to the chairs at the breakfast table on the terrace, pops of pastel shades permeate the spaces—a playful contrast to the black lava stone walls and terracotta floors.

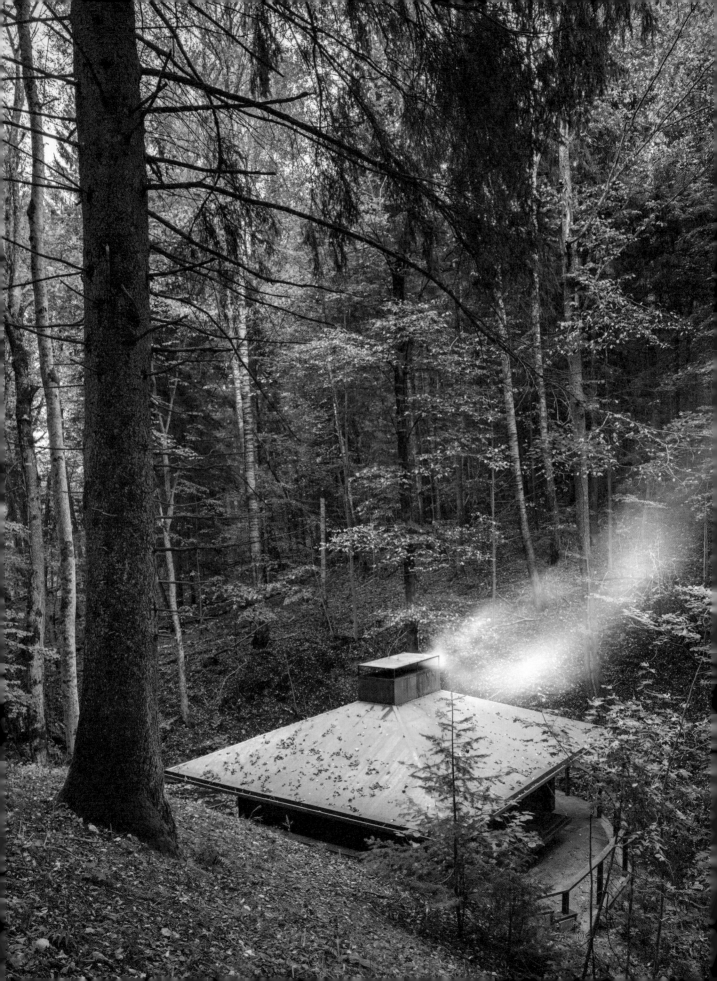

CLEANSE MIND AND BODY IN A TRADITIONAL *PIRTS* EXPERIENCE IN RURAL LATVIA

Ziedlejas
Sigulda, Latvia

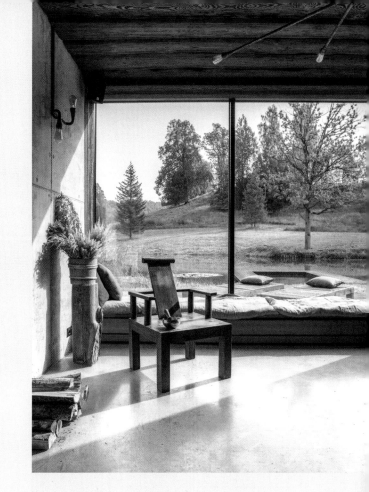

This nature spa builds on the LATVIAN SAUNA TRADITION and offers relaxing, personal BATHING SESSIONS in which each guest undergoes a range of therapies using warm air and besoms surrounded by fragrant plants.

Operating year-round, the Ziedlejas nature spa is surrounded by meadows, ponds, and forests not far from the Gauja National Park in Sigulda, Latvia. A quiet, tranquil spot, there is little to disturb the peace other than the wind in the trees and intermittent bird-song. The overall concept of the resort was inspired by local customs and beliefs. The materials used and the services provided were chosen with the aim of keeping Latvian traditions alive and adapting them to modern standards.

Guests here are invited to undergo a traditional *pirts* bathing session in one of the retreat's unique saunas. The bright Glass Sauna has one fully glazed wall, but is built into a slope to offer privacy. It has decking on which to relax and a nearby pond for swimming and cooling off. *Pirts* sessions inside center on local materials such as wood, flax, and medicinal and meadow plants—materials associated with traditional Latvian sauna culture. The Smoke Sauna is in a forest hollow, beneath a gray fir tree and close to a stream. Darker and more primitive than the Glass Sauna, its silence and proximity to nature offer guests a more authentic, ancient experience. This is the place to undergo a more personal, dedicated sauna session aimed at healing both mind and body. With its unique round shape

OPPOSITE Deep in the woods, the Smoke Sauna offers guests an authentic experience based on ancient traditions, and it has a genuinely mystical air about it.

151

and wool-covered walls, the Wool Sauna is accessed via a wooden bridge and offers a calm, meditative, warming experience. The wool wall cladding is said to have a healing effect due to its lanolin content. Outside the sauna is a tub for cooling off.

Sauna sessions are administered by one of the center's 15 professional sauna masters, and lasts around three to four hours. Each one aims to free not only the physical body, but also the mental and spiritual body, bringing greater clarity of mind. Treatments include body scrubs, swatting with besoms, head massages, and honey-based body rubs.

Guests achieve a state of deep relaxation thanks to the effects of herbal aromatherapy and the hot and cold sauna treatments. Sauna master Inese Mālniece says, "Each sauna ritual is like a unique adventure where the power of rhythm, smell, taste, and touch come together to awaken all senses, bringing pleasure, joy, and a deep awareness of life."

In addition to the regular sessions, the spa offers dedicated *pirts* rituals— focusing on

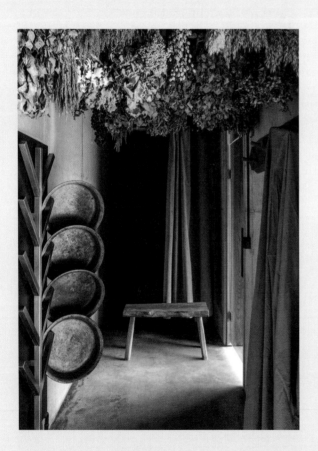

Guests are invited to undergo a traditional *pirts* bathing session in one of the retreat's unique saunas.

ABOVE Bunches of dried herbs and flowers hang from the ceiling in the entranceway to the Glass Sauna. OPPOSITE A *pirts* ritual taking place in the Wool Sauna. The plants used are local to the area and are chosen for their sensual and restorative properties.

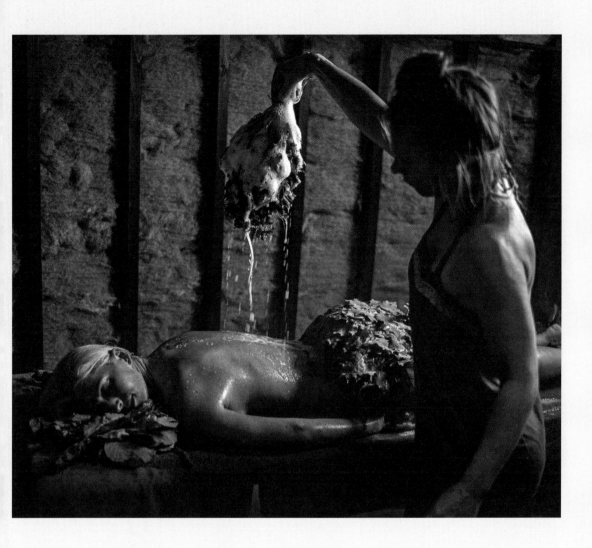

a birthday, for example, a time of year, or the healing of psycho-emotional trauma. Following each *pirts* session, guests are pampered with a special tea, fruit, and home-baked bread.

Also in the grounds at Ziedlejas are four Glass Rooms—small houses for relaxation and overnight stays. Detached from everyday life and without access to the internet, guests are left to enjoy the quiet of this rural location and to establish their own deep connection with nature. Spending a little time here to prepare for a *pirts* session and to clear the mind and body of stress enhances the whole experience, helping each guest to feel more harmonized with their sauna master.   ∗

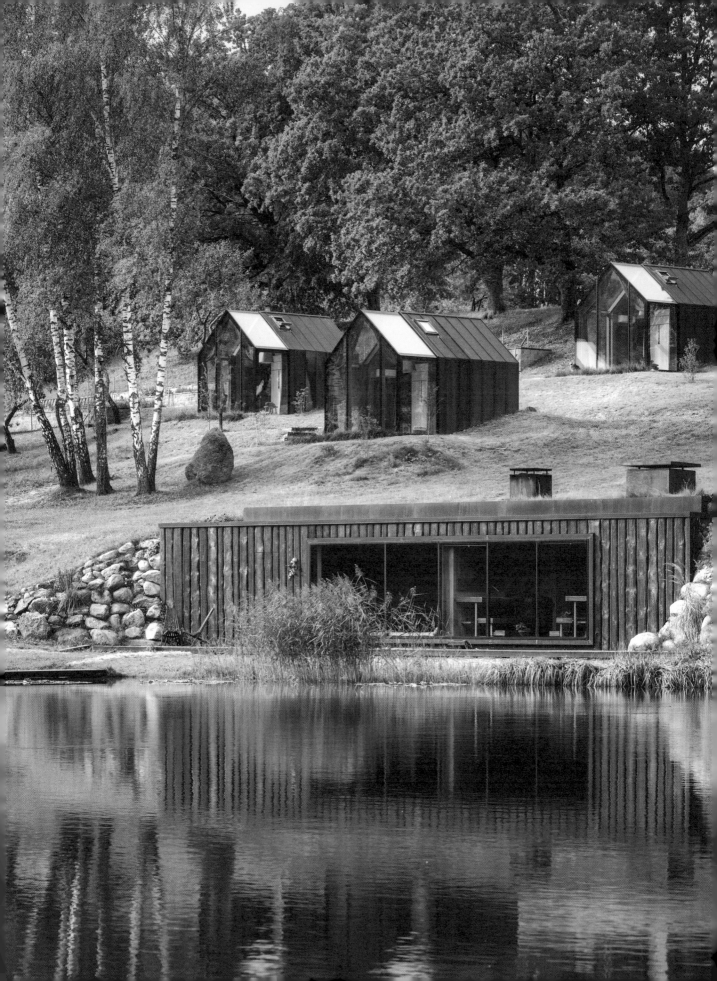

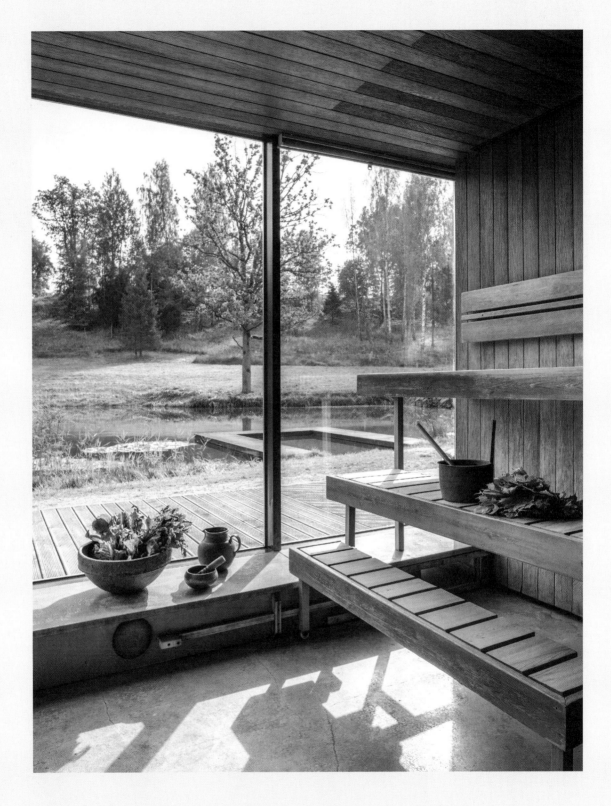

OPPOSITE The Glass Sauna, which is half-buried in the hillside, with the Glass Rooms on the slopes beyond.
ABOVE The sauna beds inside the Glass Sauna. Outside is a large pond with a small pier where guests can swim in the cool water following their *pirts* session.

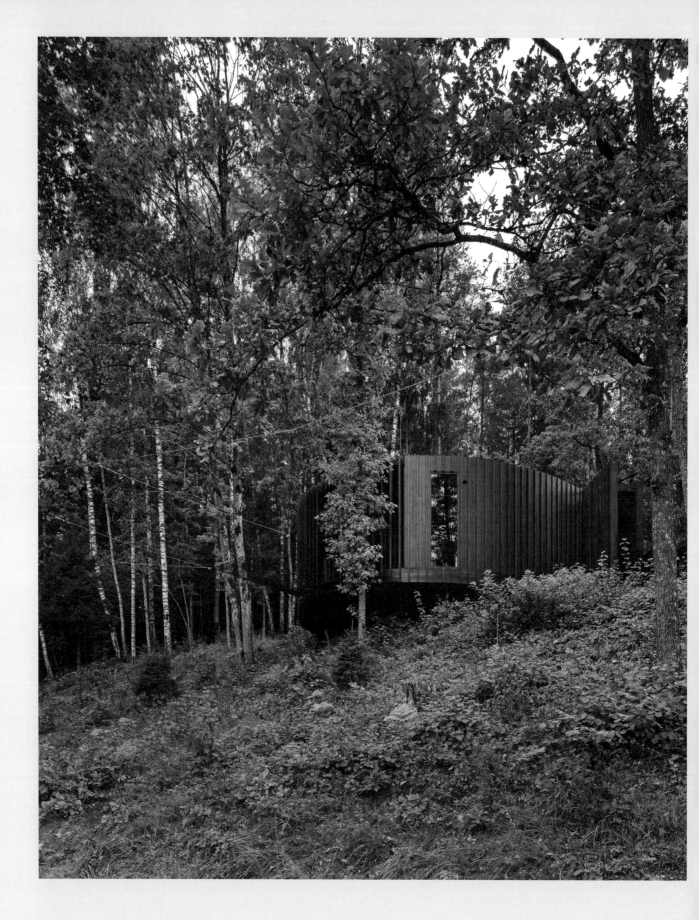

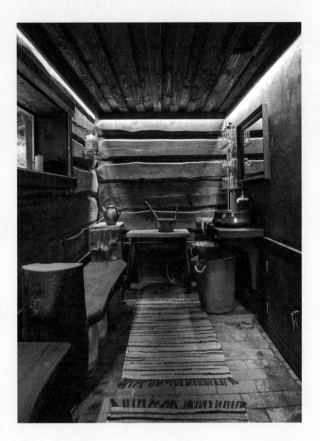
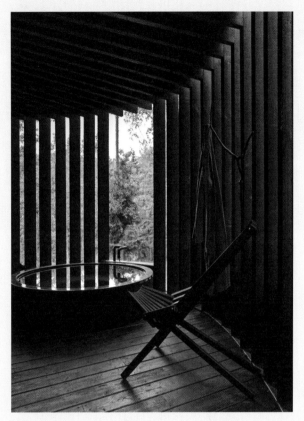

OPPOSITE AND ABOVE Dark and intimate, the Wool Sauna is nestled in the forest. Accessed via a spiraling bridge,
it has a fairy-tale feel to it. Inside lies a generous circular space with the sauna rocks at the center. There is a cooling-off
tub just outside and guests can air-dry afterward in netting suspended among the trees.

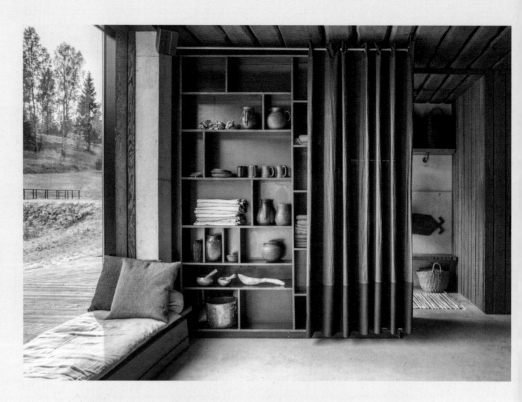

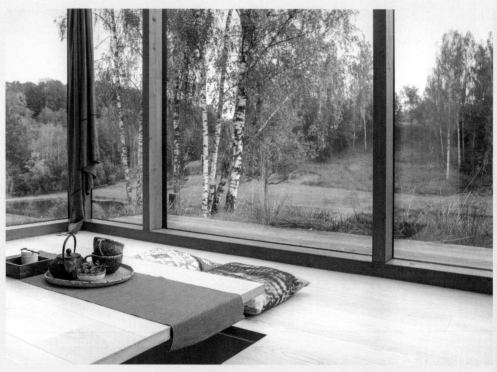

ABOVE The glass-fronted guest rooms are large enough to accommodate two adults and two children and make clever use of the space, with kids' beds in the loft, a fold-up adult bed, and a Japanese-style table that can be raised or lowered as needed.

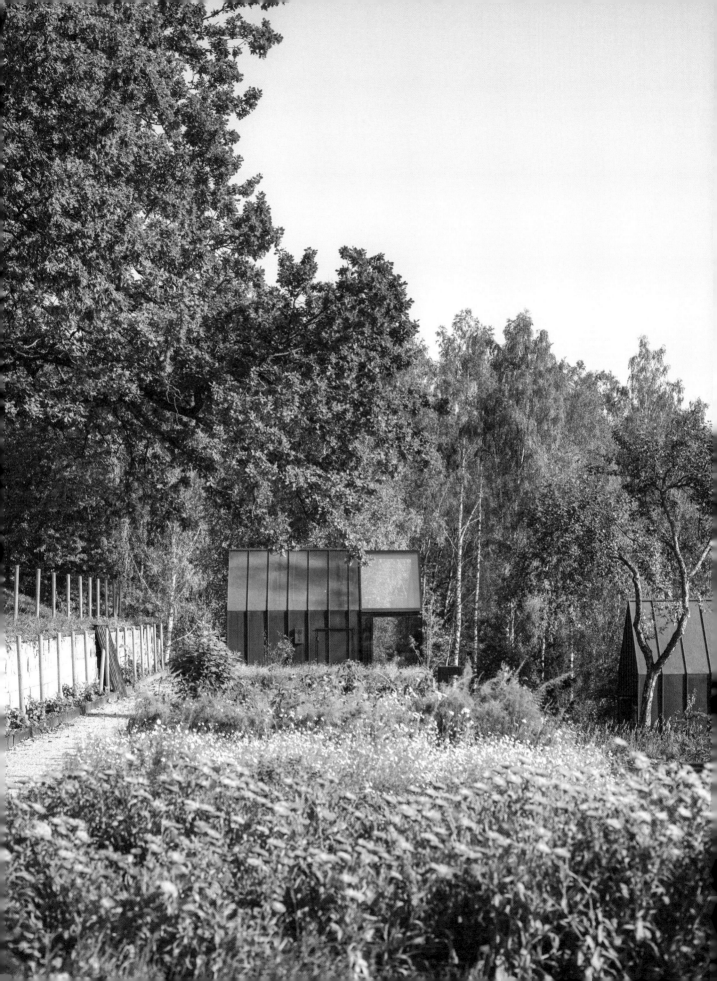

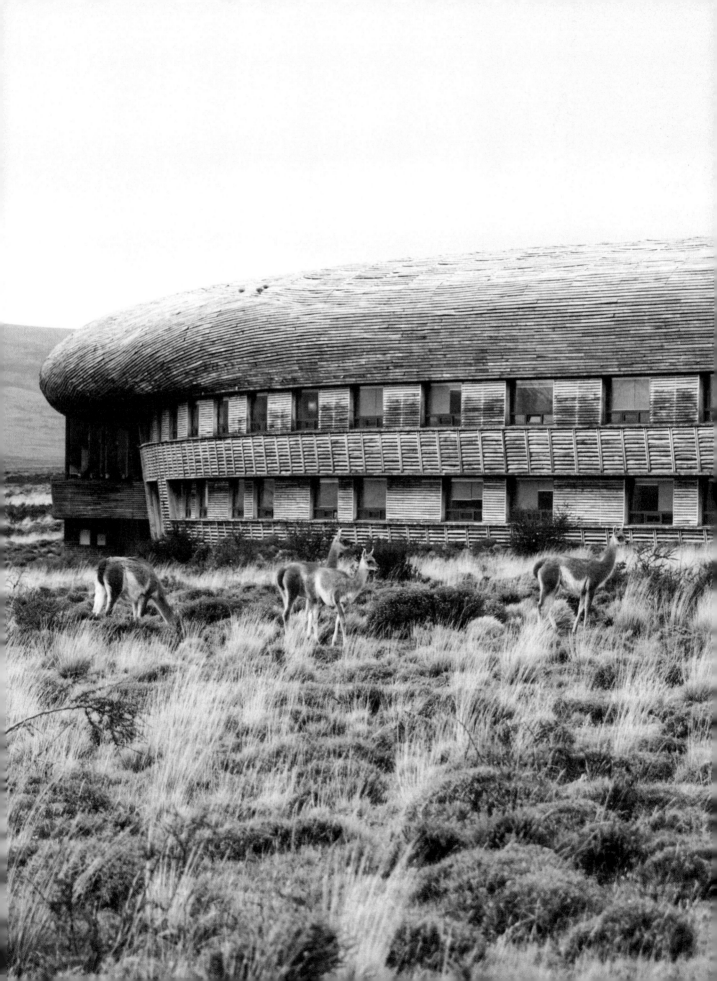

Tierra Patagonia
Torres del Paine, Chile

A WELLNESS SPA IN WHICH GUESTS FOSTER AN INTIMATE RELATIONSHIP WITH THE LAND

Whether bathing in their room, relaxing in the pool, or trekking across the landscape beyond, guests at this spa resort become immersed in their NATURAL SURROUNDINGS from the moment they arrive.

The Tierra Patagonia eco-luxury lodge overlooks Torres del Paine National Park, a raw landscape on Chile's southernmost tip, famous for its three sculptural peaks (the *torres,* or towers, for which the park is named) pine and lenga beech forests, and mirror-surfaced glacial lakes. Open from October to April—the warmest months of the year—the lodge offers an all-inclusive retreat that allows guests to explore the natural environment on the one hand while relaxing and unwinding in the hotel spa on the other. The hotel's aim is to "offer an integrated and balanced travel experience that encourages guests to discover the area and its people's inherent beauty." With architecture inspired inside and out by the local terrain, the hotel feels like a natural part of the Patagonian landscape. The lodge itself is an organic, curvaceous building clad entirely in washed lenga beech wood—a common choice among the vernacular buildings of the region.

Inside, the rooms combine wood finishes with whitewashed walls and huge picture windows that look out across the dynamic landscape. The lodge has 40 guest rooms and suites, all simply furnished and with sheepskin rugs and handmade throws for comfort, plus an in-room luxe bath from which guests can contemplate the great outdoors while taking an herbal soak.

At the heart of the complex is the Uma Spa. *Uma* means water in the Aymara language and here guests can while away the hours relaxing in a heated indoor pool, complete with hydro-massage and water jets. They also have an outdoor hot tub, a steam room, and a dry sauna at their disposal. The spa has floor-to-ceiling windows ensuring that guests feel a constant connection to the natural world.

OPPOSITE The organic design of the lodge has the least possible impact on the natural landscape. The lenga wood cladding will take on silver hues as it ages.

A three-night minimum stay at the hotel includes a generous all-inclusive program of full-board accommodation, one full-day or two half-day excursions exploring the wilds of Patagonia, and use of the spa facilities. Activities include gentle walks, hikes, and a photography tour, and guests can also explore by bike, on horseback, or by kayak. For those looking for a little more indulgence, an extensive list of facials, massages, body wraps, scrubs, and alternative therapies are also available. Come mealtime, dishes reflect the regional cuisine, focusing on hearty stews and slow-cooked soups, and wherever possible produce is sourced from local smallholdings.   ＊

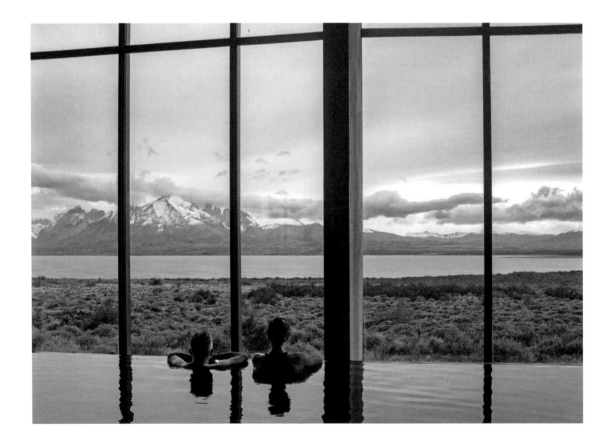

ABOVE The indoor pool is a particular highlight of the spa. Bathing in this glass-paneled sanctuary, guests have the most amazing view of the mountain landscape outside. It is not unusual to see Patagonian wildlife going about its business, oblivious to any human activity nearby.

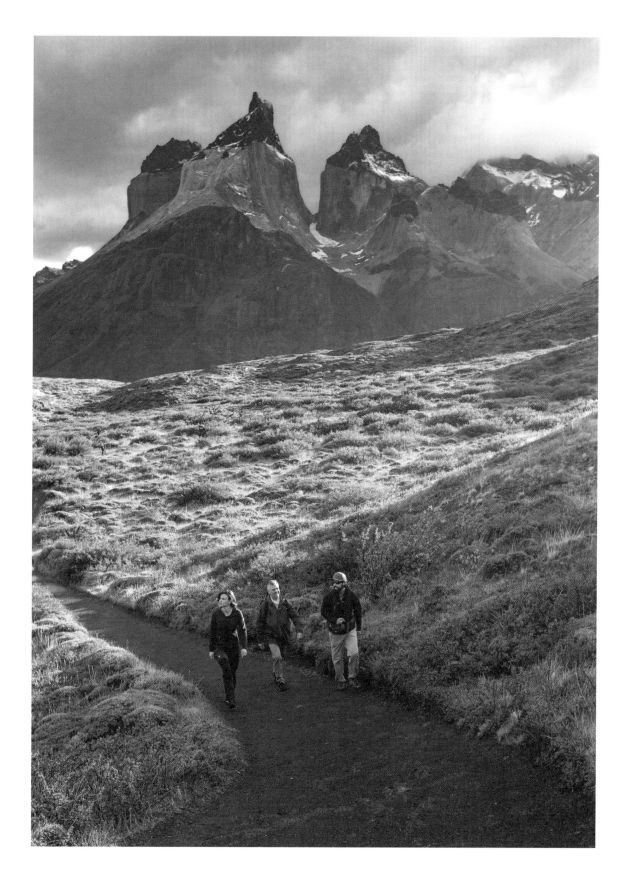

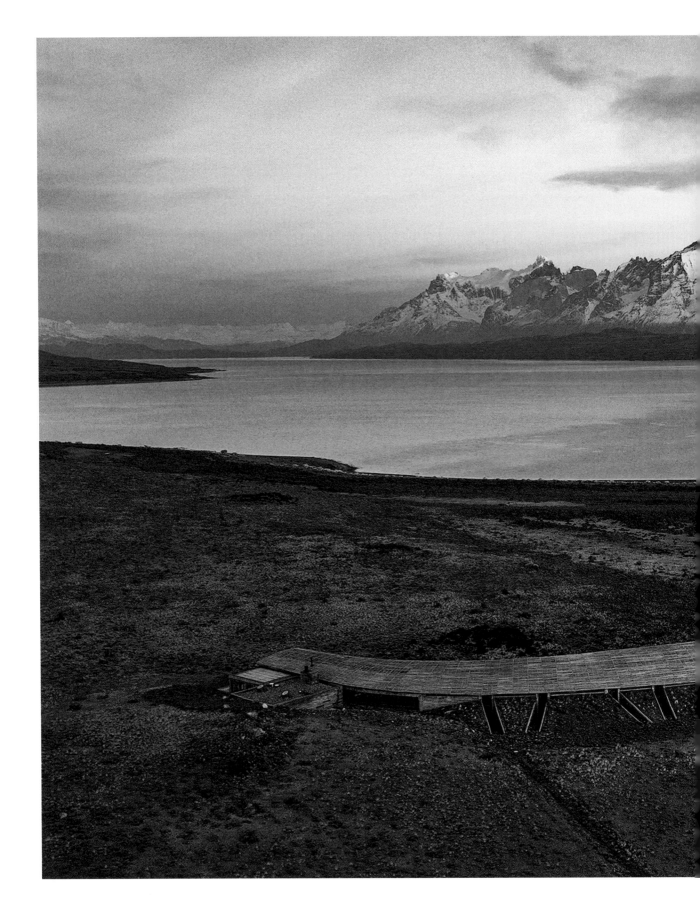

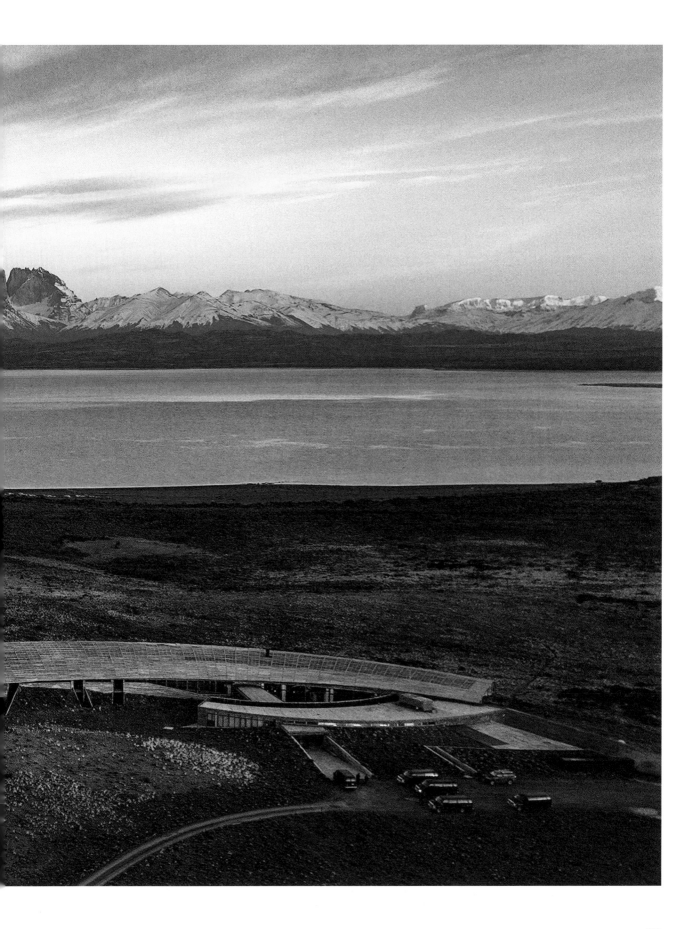

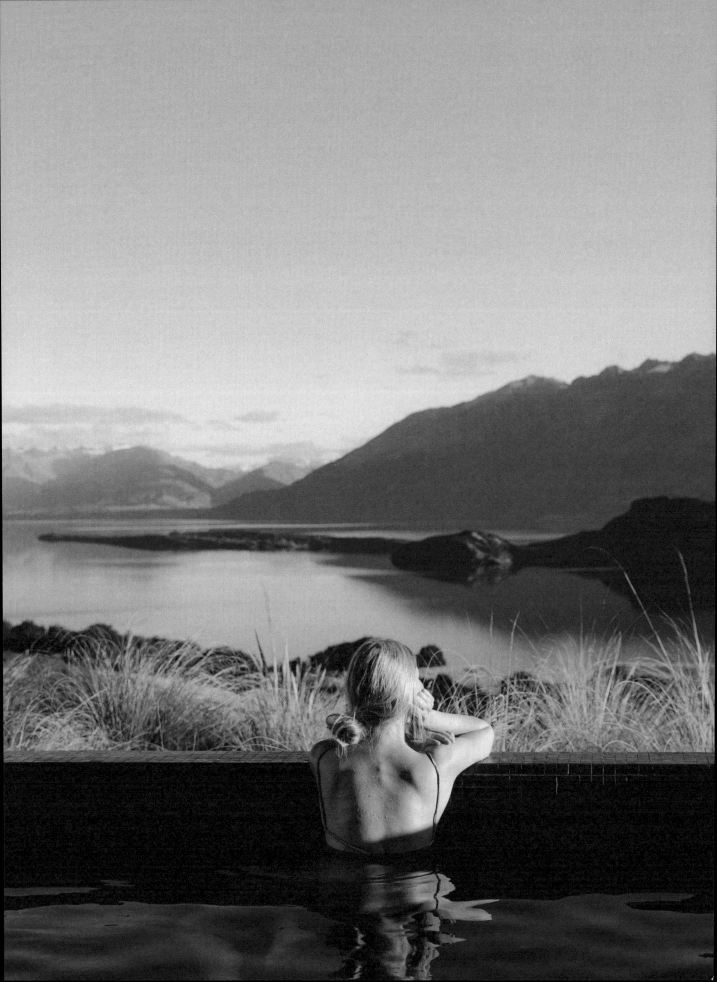

Aro Ha
Glenorchy, New Zealand

SWITCHING OFF FROM TECHNOLOGY IN THE SOUTHERN ALPS OF NEW ZEALAND

A retreat at this LUXURY SPA *addresses all aspects of natural health—guests leave leaner, stronger, and more flexible, and with a calmer, clearer, more* PRESENT STATE OF MIND.

The Aro Ha luxury spa resort is in the heart of the Southern Alps of New Zealand. It offers a mindful retreat program designed to help guests explore the human spirit through discovery, challenge, and adventure, and to nurture relationships with themselves, their families, and their environment. Guests are encouraged to develop an understanding of what it means to live a connected, balanced life and to improve their physical, emotional, and spiritual health through the cultivation of new daily habits.

A sustainable property overlooking Lake Wakatipu on New Zealand's South Island, Aro Ha comprises a main activity hub surrounded by state-of-the-art log cabins for guests to sleep in—two rooms per cabin with a shared bathroom. The rooms are simply arranged with natural furnishings and have views over the lake and across miles of rugged countryside. At the heart of the resort is a welcome lodge with a communal living room and a dining room in which guests gather around a large table.

The property also has a yoga studio and a spa pavilion with several massage rooms and two saunas. Just outside the pavilion are a hot tub and an ice-cold plunge pool. Among the unique features of the Ara Ha resort are the permaculture gardens that provide up to 45 percent of the food served at mealtimes, with menus focused on seasonal produce to create gluten-free, plant-based dishes designed to detoxify, rejuvenate, and heal.

The resort recommends a stay of five nights to make the most of its daily wellness program, and carefully balances group and solo activities so that guests enjoy both solitude and community. Guests can expect to start their

OPPOSITE A guest looks out across Lake Wakatipu from the resort's outdoor pool. Built into the terrace, this cold pool is the perfect spot to refresh after a sauna session at the spa.

days in the yoga studio, watching the sun rise over the mountains, before enjoying a well-balanced, nourishing breakfast in the dining hall. They can then explore one of several subalpine trails, immersing themselves in nature and experiencing its transformative power. Throughout the day various mindfulness practices interweave with activities that range from cooking classes to functional strength training. Later there is time for guests to unwind with a sauna before receiving their daily massage.

Each retreat is all-inclusive, with daily massage, all food and beverages, guided hikes, workshops, and transport to and from the retreat from the nearest major city, Queenstown, as standard. Additional treatments are available and include Reiki, osteopathy, and women's well-being.   ✻

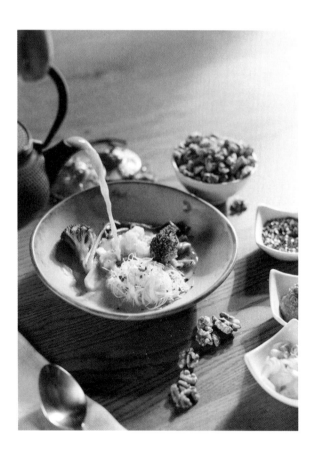

ABOVE Come mealtime, dishes are nutrient-dense, gluten-free, and full of variety and flavor. The retreat center prides itself on finding new ways to prepare vegetables, and each meal is designed to detoxify, rejuvenate, heal, and delight.

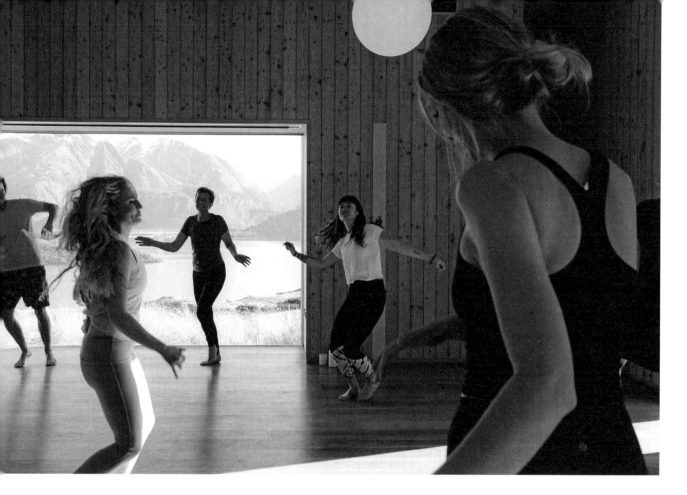

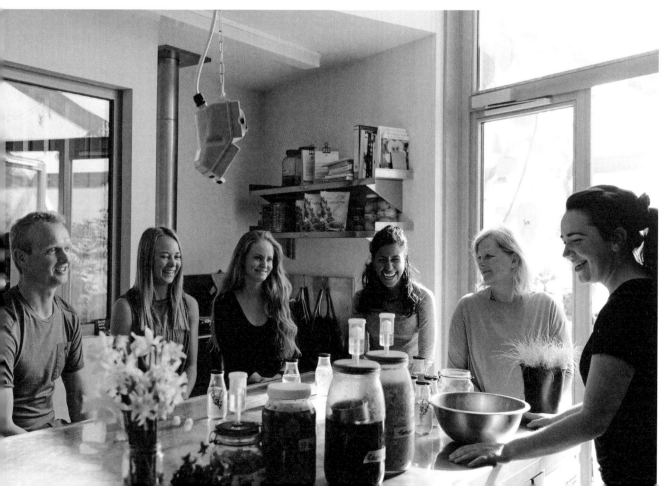

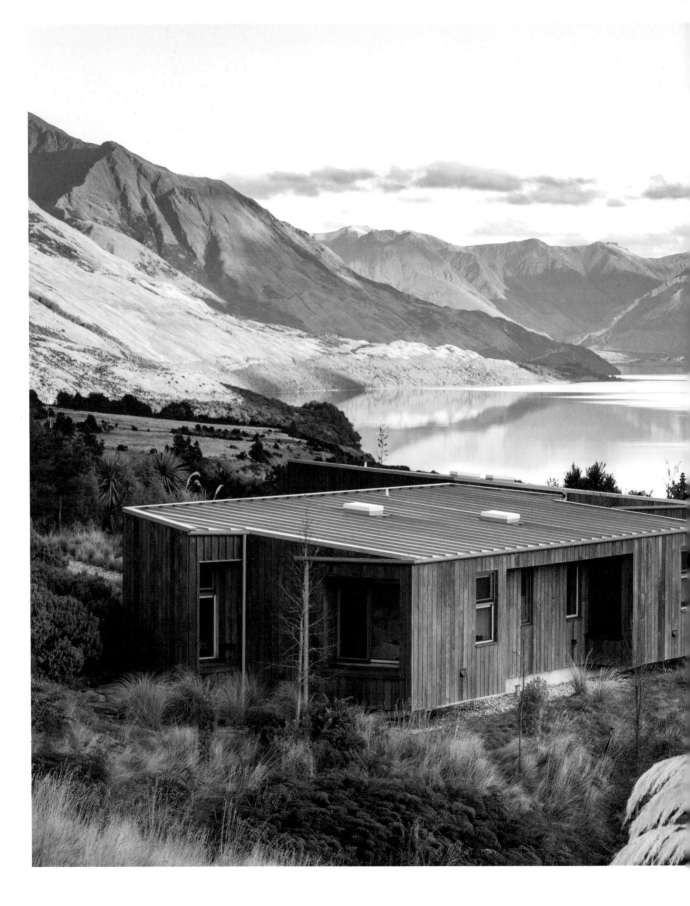

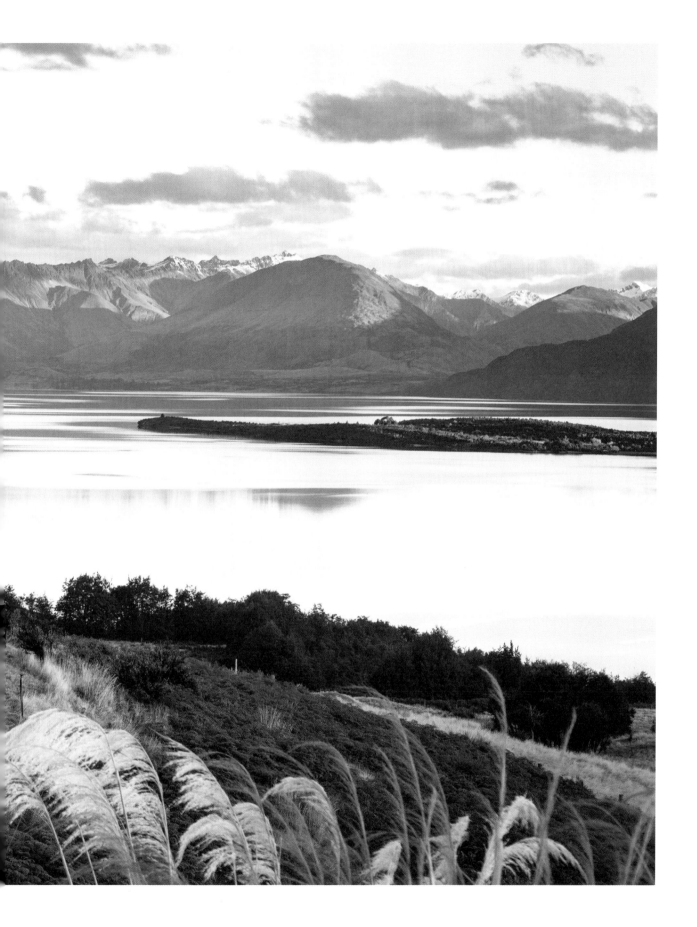

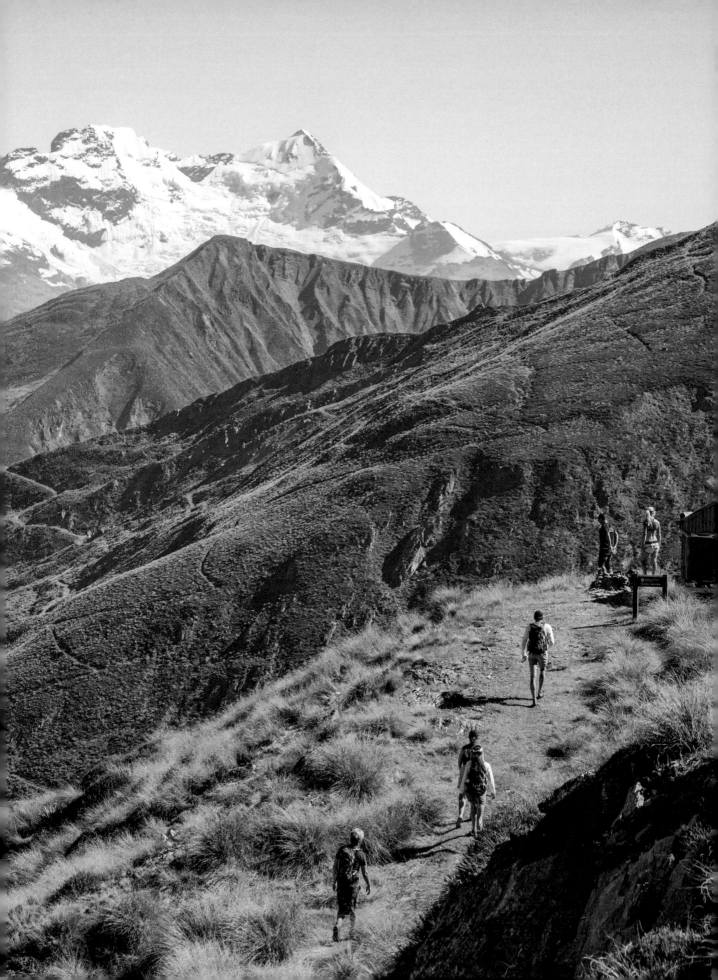

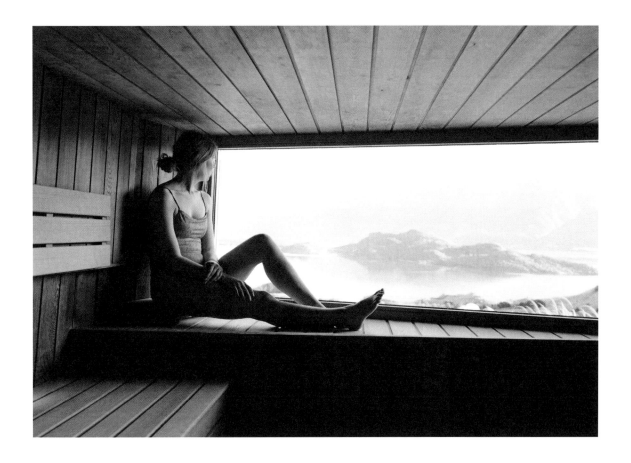

OPPOSITE Restorative hikes across the wild South Island terrain are on the itineraries of some of the retreats at this resort.
ABOVE A picture window in the Finnish sauna perfectly frames the vast rugged landscape outside.

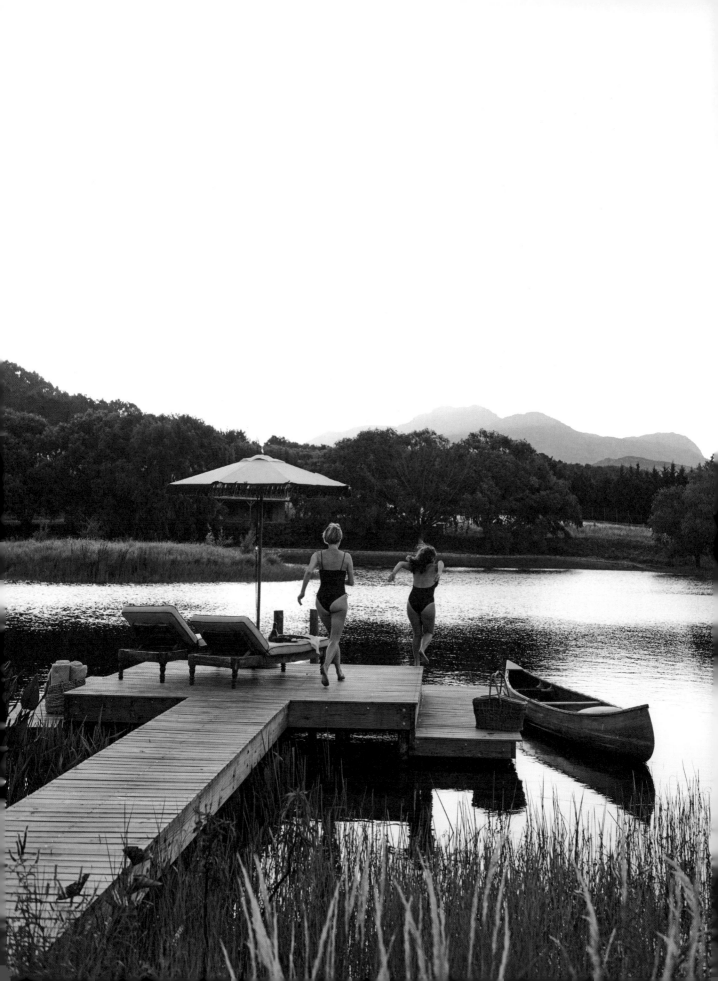

Sterrekopje Farm
Franschhoek, Western Cape, South Africa

A VOYAGE OF DEEP SERENITY IN THE FOOTHILLS OF SOUTH AFRICA'S MAJESTIC FRANSCHHOEK MOUNTAINS

Guided by ANCESTRAL WISDOM and a conscious way of living, luxurious Sterrekopje Farm exists to REGENERATE earth, body, and soul through its daily offering of Farmhouse Rhythms and Bathhouse Rituals.

An hour's drive from Cape Town, in South Africa, lies a 125-acre (50-hectare) biodiverse, regenerative farm in the foothills of the Franschhoek mountains. Sterrekopje, a "soulful sanctuary of healing," is owned by a family of holistic practitioners and offers guests a carefully curated program of treatments, ancient philosophies, and healing practices in the most beautiful, natural surroundings. From morning yoga to the daily harvest and from pottery classes to evening sound baths, movement, creativity, and play are gently woven into the fabric of the farm's daily rhythm.

Eleven guest rooms are dotted around the estate, with several in the main farmhouse and others tucked away in the gardens. Classed variously as Intimate Sanctuaries, Abundant Sanctuaries, or Rejuvenating Suites, each has been designed for rest and rejuvenation. Everything here is carefully designed to encourage deep restorative sleep and inspire contemplation and creativity. And no two rooms are the same.

Activities at the retreat fall into two groups: Farmhouse Rhythms and Bathhouse Rituals. Among the former are a range of painting, drawing, and pottery classes held in the farmhouse atelier. The latter include cleansing rituals, movement classes such as yoga and qigong, and a range of healing meditative practices.

When it comes to the daily harvest, the estate has 17 acres (7 hectares) of productive garden, healing herb gardens, and orchards in which more than 60 varieties of indigenous and heritage plants are grown. The owners live by a philosophy of eating seasonally, respectfully, and with as little waste as possible.

OPPOSITE Taking the plunge. Guests have several options for wild swimming in pools, ponds, and dams dotted around the retreat's extensive gardens.

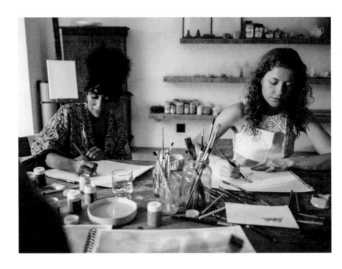

They grow, harvest, and raise most of their ingredients and source and collaborate with other local artisans and producers for the rest. Mealtimes take place at the large communal table in the farmhouse kitchen.

Four times a year, the farm also hosts a Wise Women Retreat that encourages guests to build deeper connections with their feminine power and to embark on a gentle and joyful journey of self-remembering and reclamation. There are also late-season retreats for families.

Making the most of the warmer seasons, the farm operates from mid-October to mid-July, closing for just a couple months in winter so that the farm and its family can rest and rejuvenate. Guests can stay for a minimum of two nights, but to truly benefit from the Sterrekopje way and pace of life, five nights or more are recommended.   *

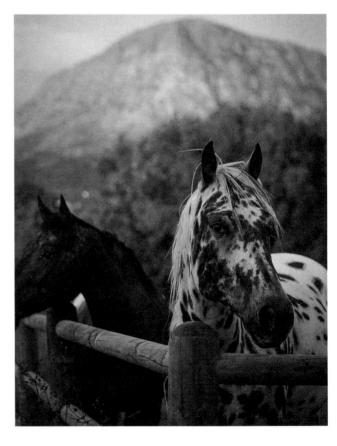

TOP The old farmhouse is home to the main activity rooms and communal space including the kitchen/bakery, library, and the atelier. OPPOSITE The long passageway leads to the orangery—a lush conservatory tea room with a lofty ceiling and handsome hand-carved doors.

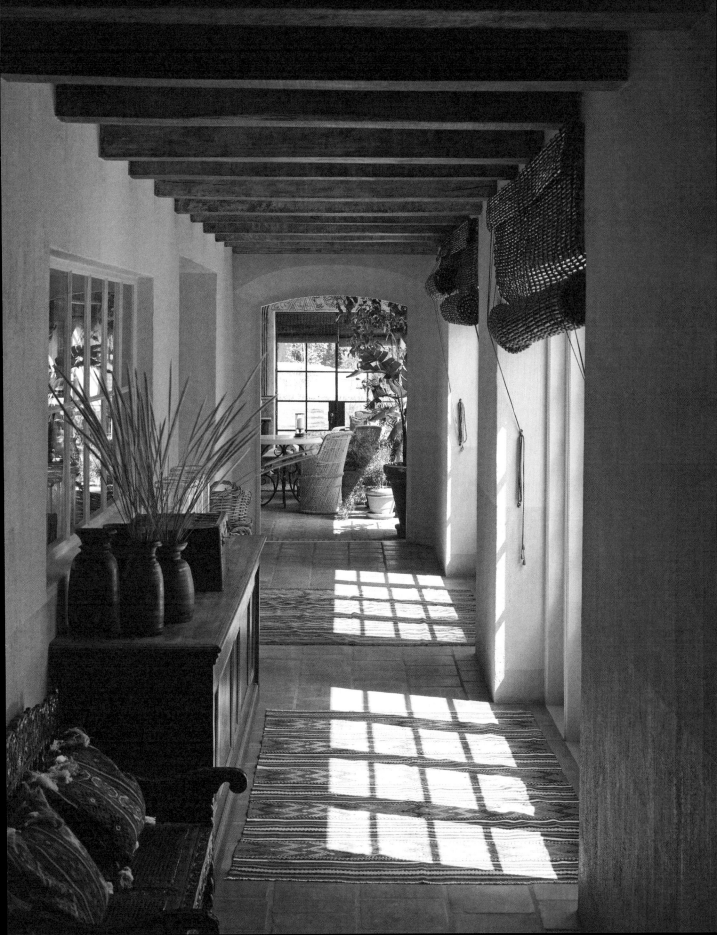

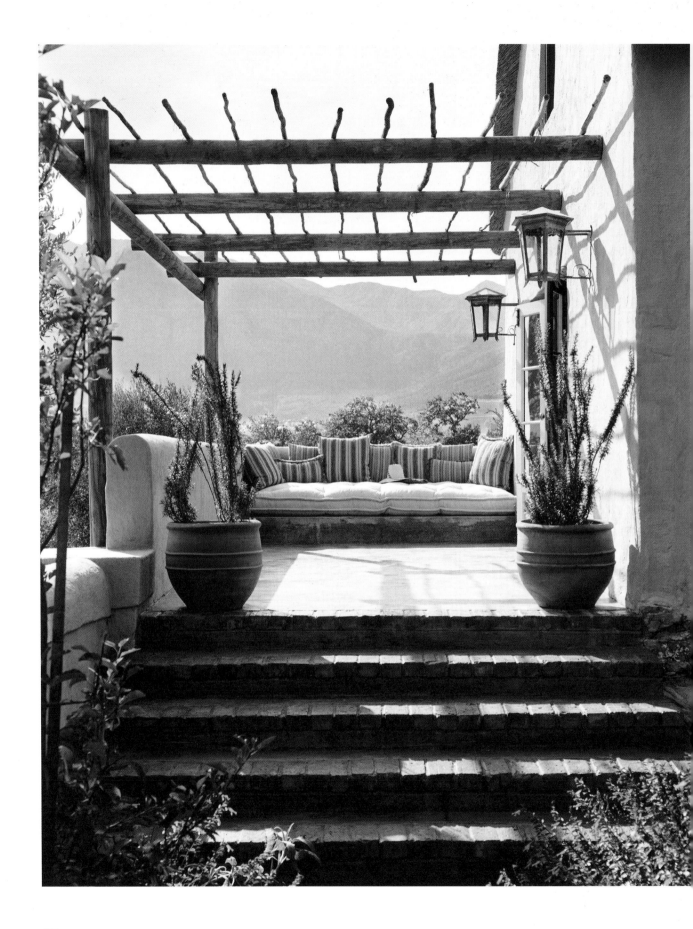

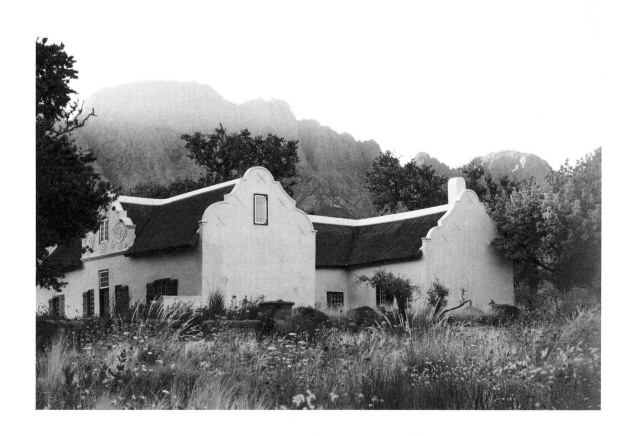

OPPOSITE Whether the private terrace adjoining a guest room or a public space outside the main farmhouse, there
are many secret nooks and sun-drenched crannies for spending time in quiet contemplation. ABOVE The main farmhouse
is surrounded by meadowland.

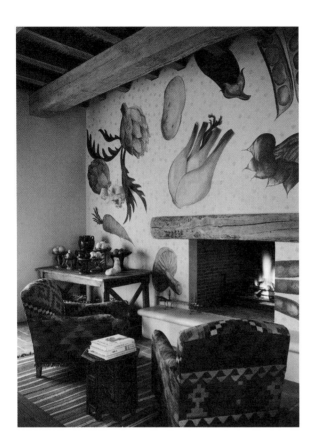
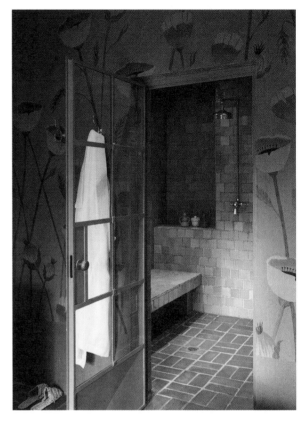

ABOVE AND OPPOSITE All of the rooms at the retreat display a rich tapestry of colors and textures, cultures, and stories. They are furnished with hand-crafted pieces and the finest soft furnishings and elaborate murals adorn many of the walls.

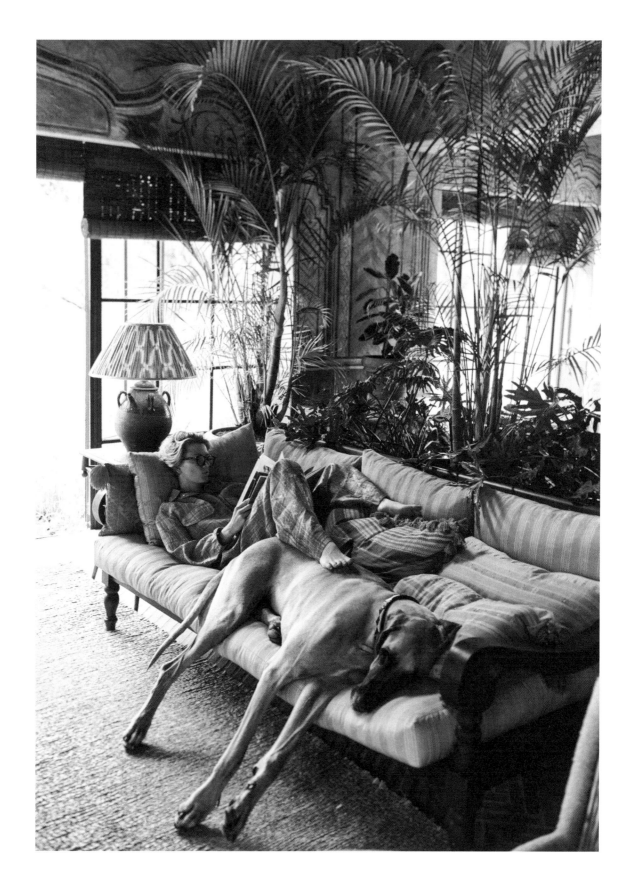

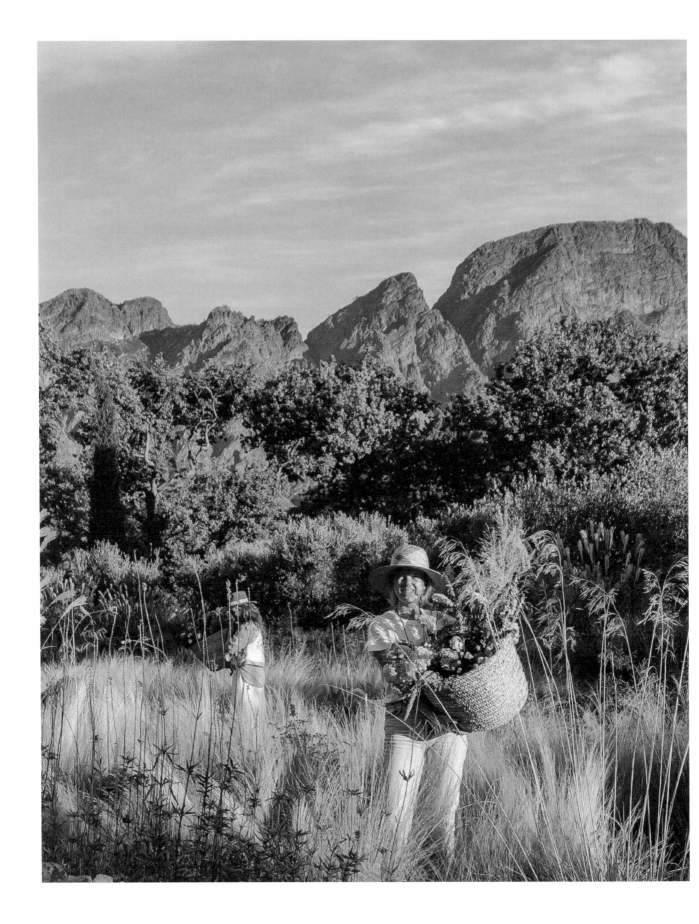

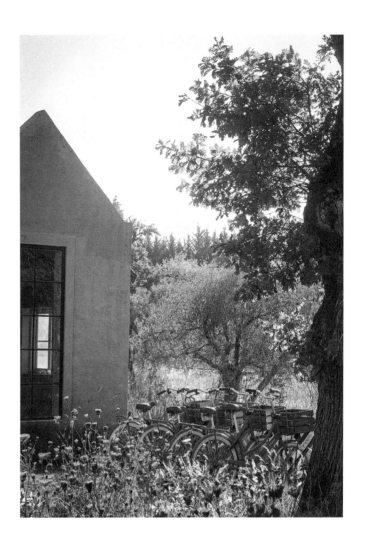

OPPOSITE AND ABOVE The retreat owners restored the farm's ancestral lands to be as fruitful and sustainable
as they were generations ago. Today, more than 100 varieties of indigenous and heritage plants grow here.

183

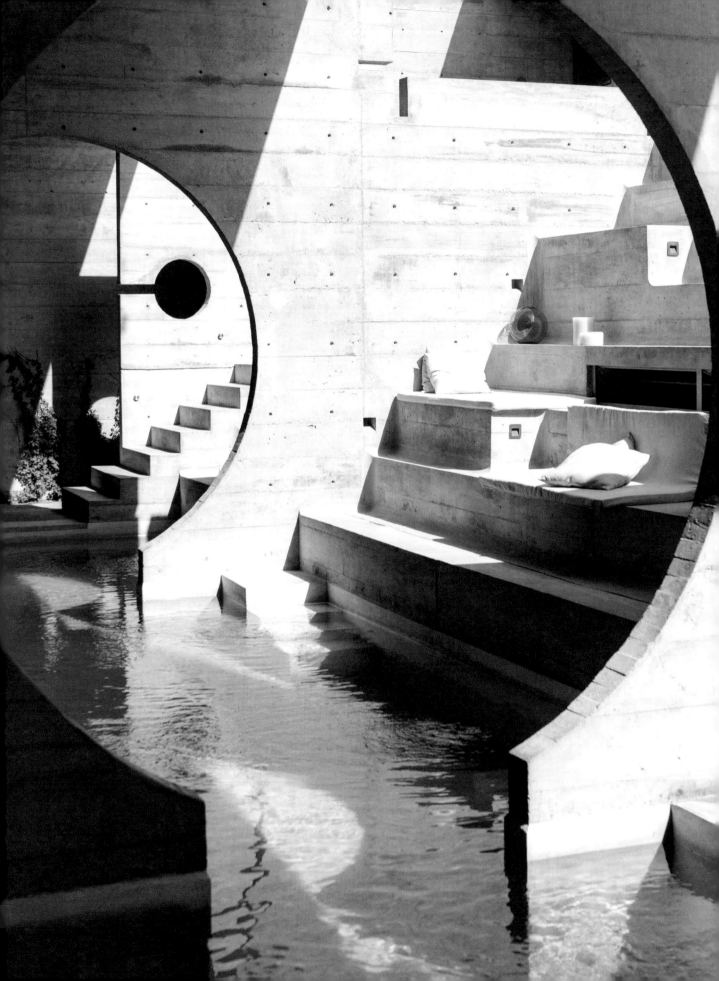

A SPACE FOR DEEP CONTEMPLATION IN A SERENE OASIS WITH OAXACAN TEMPLE VIBES

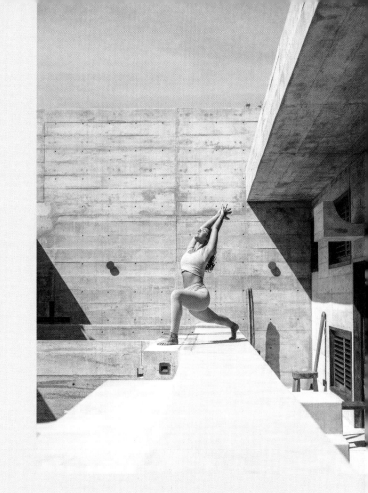

Casa TO

Oaxaca, Mexico

Surrounded by the greenery of a nearby ECOLOGICAL RESERVE and within easy walking distance of the BEACH, Casa TO harmonizes with its natural environment to create a HAVEN OF PEACE and tranquility.

Not far from the popular surfing resort of Puerto Escondido on Mexico's Pacific coast, Casa TO is a two-story boutique hotel with just nine suites. Designed by French-born, Mexico City—based architect Ludwig Godefroy, the elegant hotel is fashioned almost entirely from concrete that has been cast in situ. The guest rooms are all located on one side of the building, and they each have an external space with high walls to provide both privacy and shade from the fierce summer heat of the Mexican sun. While the six ground-floor suites have their own gardens, the three on the upper level offer terraces with outdoor baths. Inside, the rooms

are miniature sanctuaries—cool, calm, and simply furnished. Walls are left with the concrete exposed, and much of the built-in furniture, from benches and shelving to vanities and beds, is cast from the same material. Additional custom furniture is designed by local craftspeople, and colorful rugs and tapestries soften the clean, minimalist edges. There is also an abundance of potted plants. Interweaving aesthetics and functionality and emphasizing the honesty of the textures of the raw materials such as concrete, steel, clay, and wood, Godefroy has made the rooms perfect spaces for contemplation. At ground level, a swimming pool runs the

OPPOSITE The hotel's central pool is a particular highlight, designed in such a way that there are seemingly no boundaries between the inside and outside spaces.

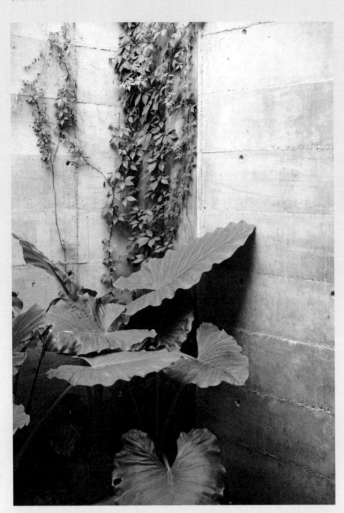

LEFT There is abundant greenery inside and out. OPPOSITE The circle motif repeats throughout the hotel. The communal lounge area flanking the pool has shallow vaulting to the roof, mirroring the circular opening, and a brick-paved floor.

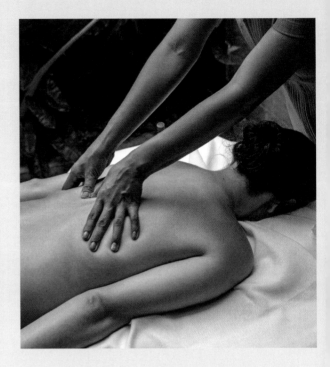

entire length of an almost cavelike public space inspired by the Yerebatan Sarayi (Basilica Cistern) of Istanbul. At intervals, the room is intersected with walls cut through with huge circular openings. On the one hand, these walls create little pockets of privacy for the guests; on the other, their openings allow for views across the hotel and out to the vegetation beyond. In the words of the hotel owner, "the interior views create an oasis enclosed by the sky, the weight of the walls, and the vegetation of climbing plants." Reminiscent of the ancient Oaxacan temples

the region is known for, stepped seating rises up from the swimming pool to connect the two floors of the hotel via a series of open spaces that allow a constant circulation of air to keep the interior cool. They lead to a rooftop where guests can enjoy views of the surrounding jungle. Also found on the rooftop is the hotel's restaurant, Glou Glou, which focuses on seasonal dishes made using local produce, washed down with a selection of organic wines.

Open all year round, the hotel offers a range of meditative experiences, including in-room

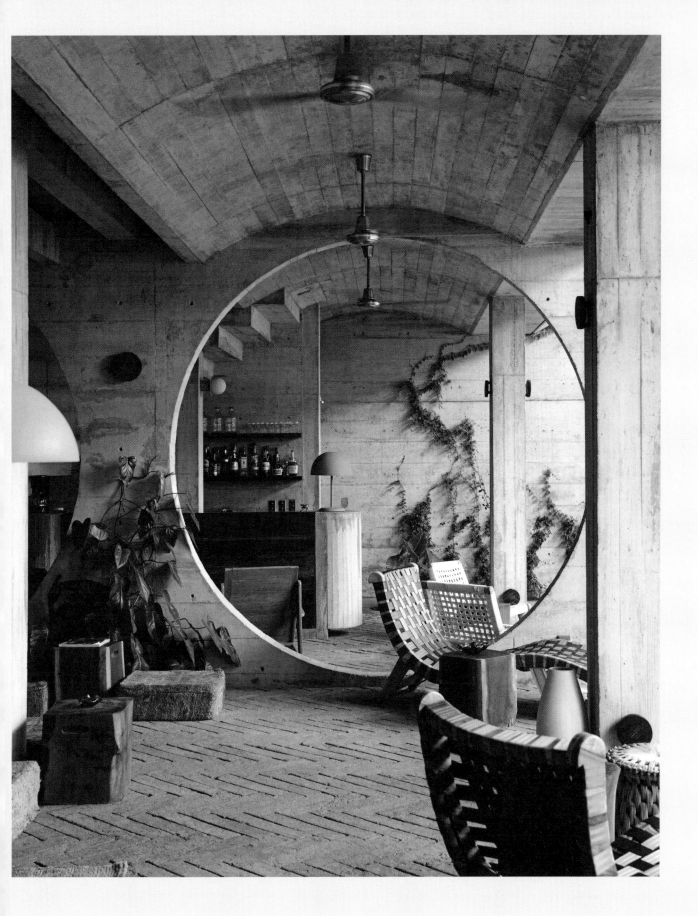

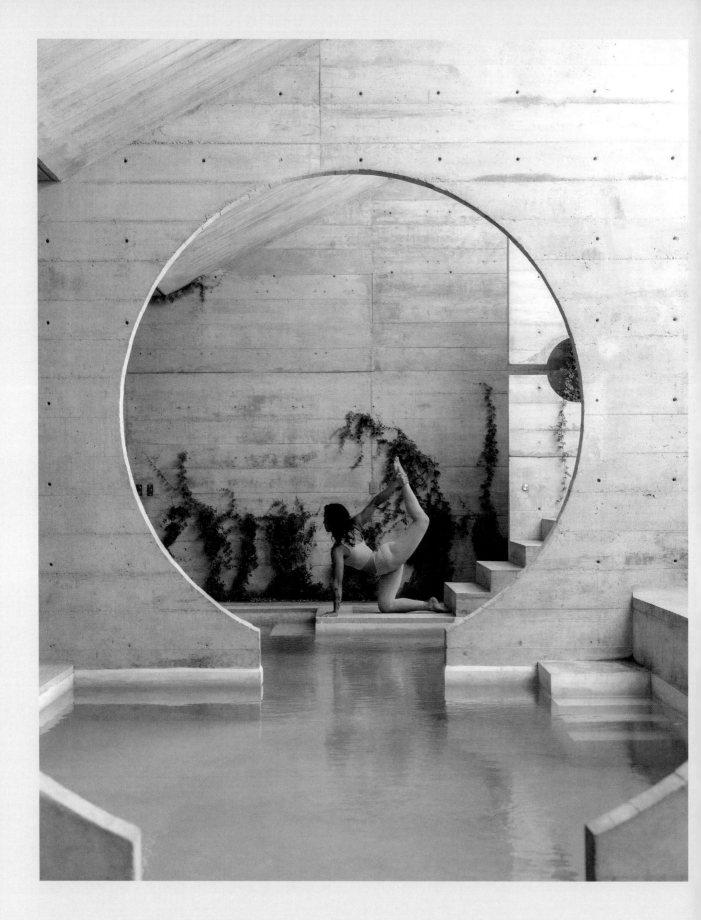

Interweaving aesthetics
and functionality, the
rooms are perfect spaces
for contemplation.

yoga and massages and trips to local thermal waters and the Lagunas de Chacahuan National Park with pristine beaches and stunning wildlife. The best weather is to be had in the months of November to April, although those who don't mind the heat will find May to September less crowded.

All rooms come with a welcome mezcal and daily breakfast at Glou Glou. For a more luxurious experience, guests can throw in airport transportation and a seven-course dinner with wine pairings.   *

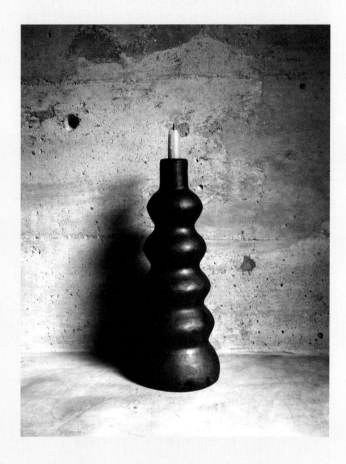

OPPOSITE The transversal walls are pierced with large, circular openings that cut through the pool serve to break up the space into smaller areas. This design feature means that guests have more privacy for practicing yoga or meditating uninterrupted by others.

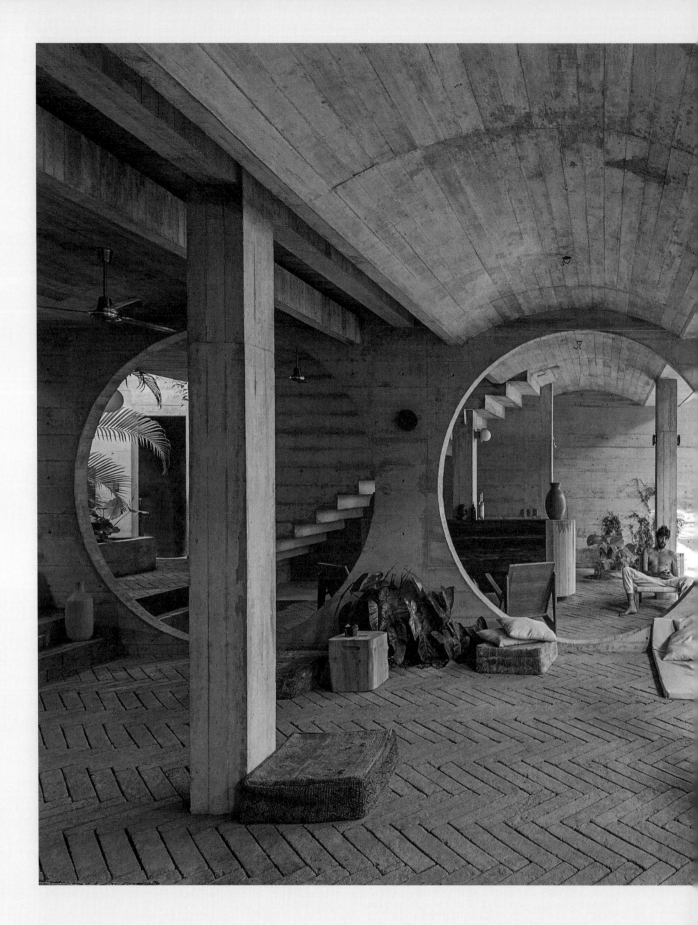

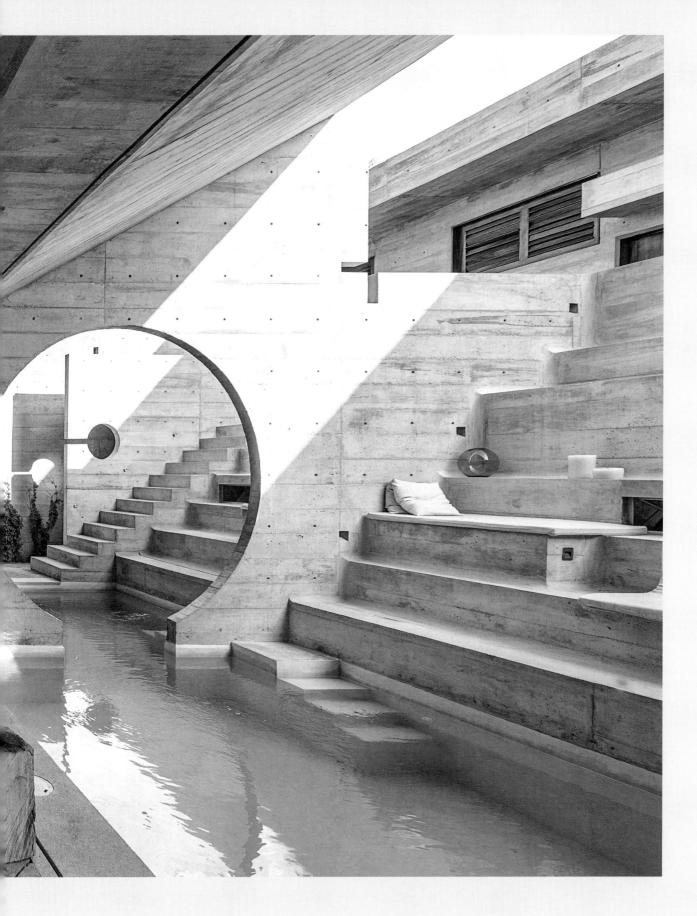

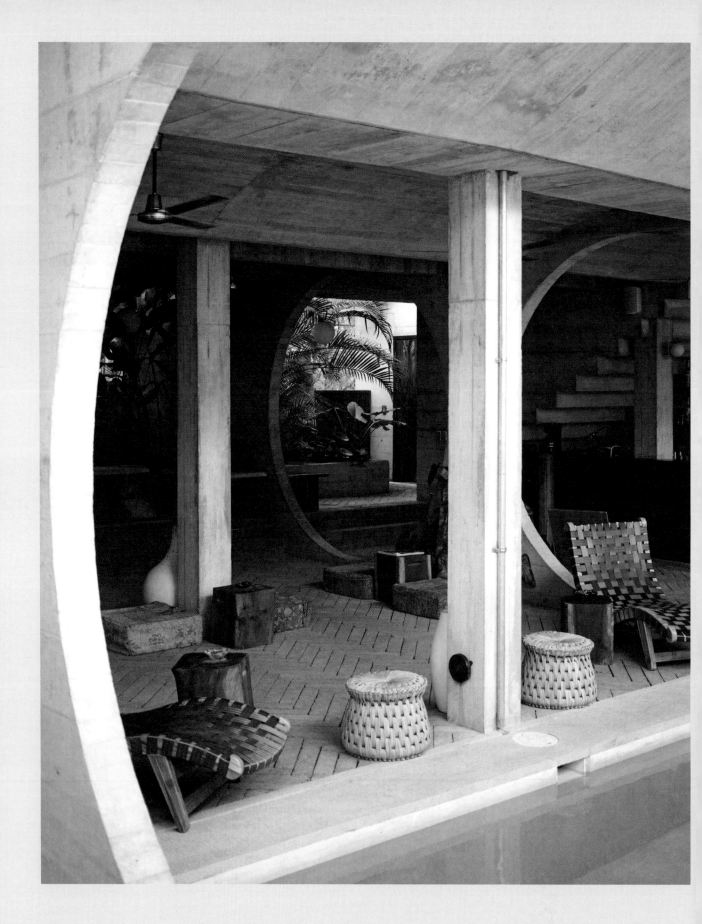

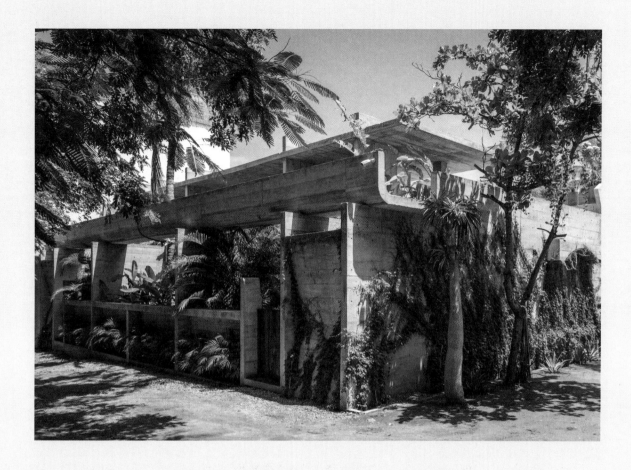

ABOVE This section of the hotel houses the guestrooms, each with their private ground-floor gardens and upper-level terraces. Numerous openings in the facade generate cross-breezes through the structure, which help to keep the interiors fresh and cool.

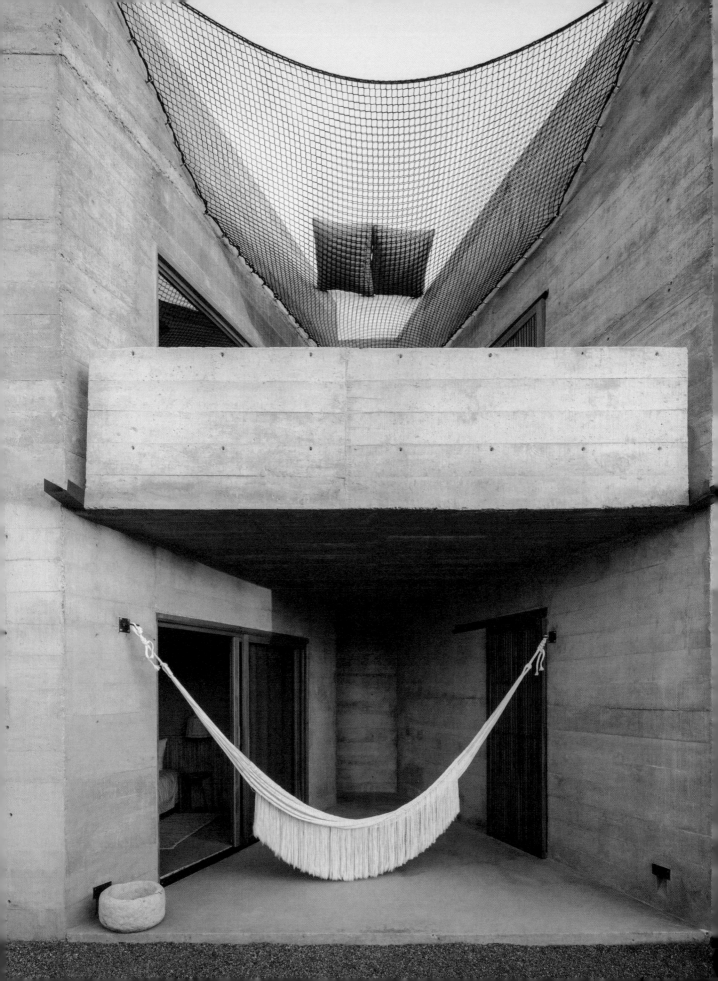

MEXICO'S PREMIERE WELLNESS-FOCUSED HOTEL EXPERIENCE, LOCATED ON THE BAJA CALIFORNIA PENINSULA

Paradero Todos Santos
Todos Santos, Mexico

At Paradero Todos Santos, guests experience everything from virgin beaches and vast farmlands to dense cacti forests, and become immersed in the region's DISTINCTIVE CULTURE, *culinary traditions, and* ANCIENT HEALING PRACTICES.

On the Baja California Peninsula in Mexico, Paradero Todos Santos, is at the luxury end of the wellness-focused hotel experience. Spread across 5 acres (2 hectares), the hotel offers wide-ranging views across the cacti-strewn Baja California Desert to the peaks of the Sierra La Laguna mountain range as well as miles of working farmland and the pristine beaches of the Pacific coast. Designed by Rubén Valdez and Yashar Yektajo, the complex itself features a 100,000-square-foot (9,000-sq-m) botanical garden and a 130-foot-long (40-m) infinity pool. Guests have their pick of 41 suites and multiple sensory offerings from the hotel's Ojo de Agua spa.

Blurring the line between outdoor and indoor living, all sanctuary-like suites have private outside spaces for revitalizing and reflecting in nature. Ground-floor suites back onto gardens equipped with an outdoor soaking tub and a hammock from which to admire the "wall" of cordon cacti beyond. Rooftop suites have panoramic decks with "star nets" in which guests can lie back and gaze at the night sky.

Exclusive experiences lie at the heart of the Paradero Todos journey, and guests would need to come for at least three days in order to fully immerse themselves in nature via a generous program of activities. These include surfing at Cerritos or San Pedrito beach, hiking and mountain biking along the bluffs of the Pacific coast, hands-on farming tutorials, and a wide range of mediation, yoga, and cooking classes. Limited to four to six guests at a time, the activities are intimate and personal.

OPPOSITE Each of the suites has a sky net or a hammock for guests to lounge in throughout their stay and gaze out across the desert by day or the stars at night.

BELOW AND OPPOSITE Inside and out, the color scheme of the property is predominantly monochromatic, based on a natural palette. All furnishings are custom-crafted and sourced locally from cities such as Guadalajara and Oaxaca—largely considered the design capitals of Mexico.

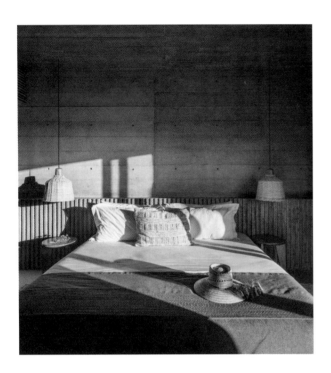

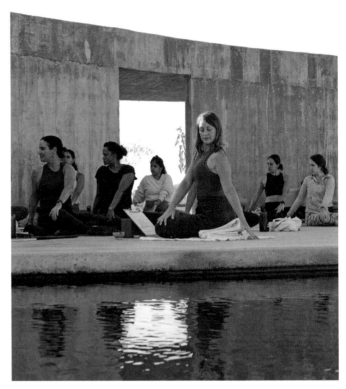

At mealtimes, guests are treated to a menu of farm-to-table cooking based on locally sourced ingredients—many of them traveling only a few steps from the on-site herb garden and 160 acres (65 hectares) of local farmland. Much of the ethos at Paradero Todos Santos stems from the desire for guests to experience a transformation of the body, mind, and spirit. All movement classes take place outside surrounded by lush greenery, the fresh salt air of the Pacific, and the warming sun. Treatments at the Ojo de Agua healing sanctuary are inspired by ancient healing practices and include a Yenekamu Ritual that combines a hot stone massage and a hip adjustment that realigns the spine and harmonizes negative emotions, and the Niparaja y Anajicondi couple's treatment, which strengthens the bond between lovers thanks to the damiana herb, which acts a natural aphrodisiac.   ✳

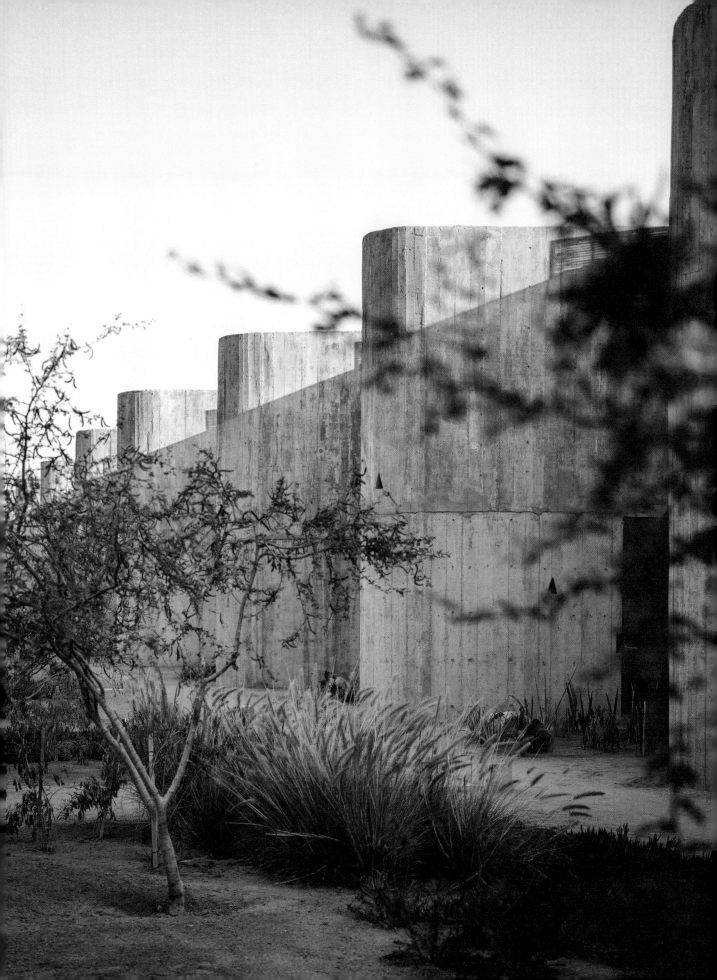

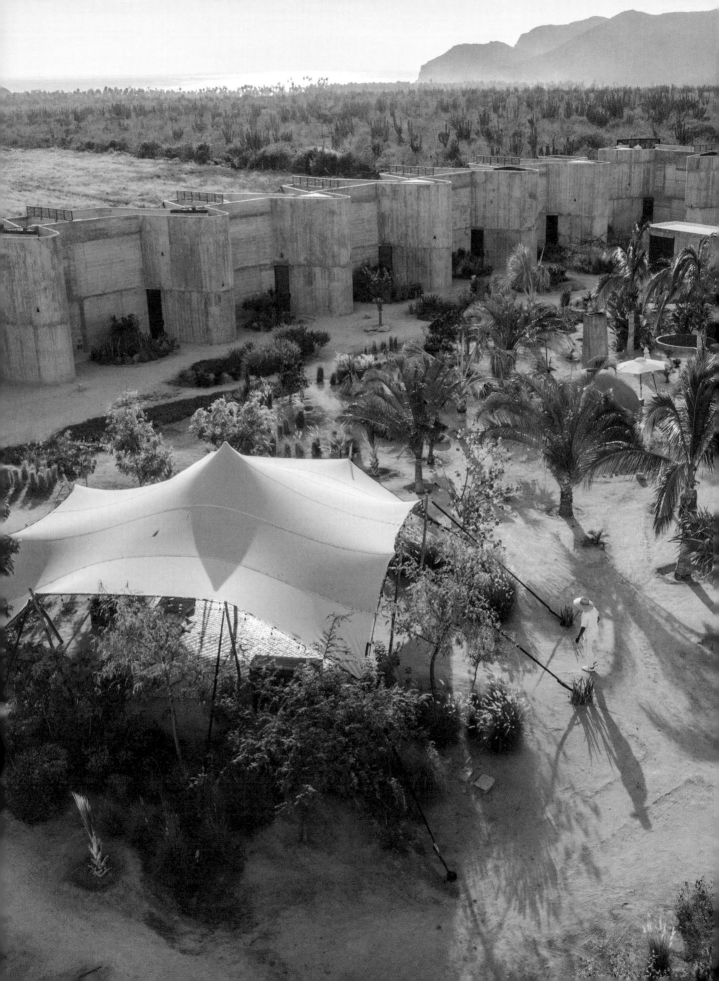

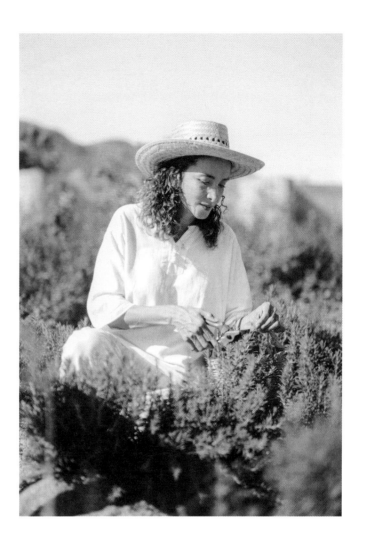

OPPOSITE The hotel suites flank two sides of a large square, which is planted with locally grown palm trees. Inside the square are the yoga *shala,* an outdoor gym, and a sweat lodge. This space is also used for outdoor cooking classes, meditation sessions, and sound healing ceremonies.

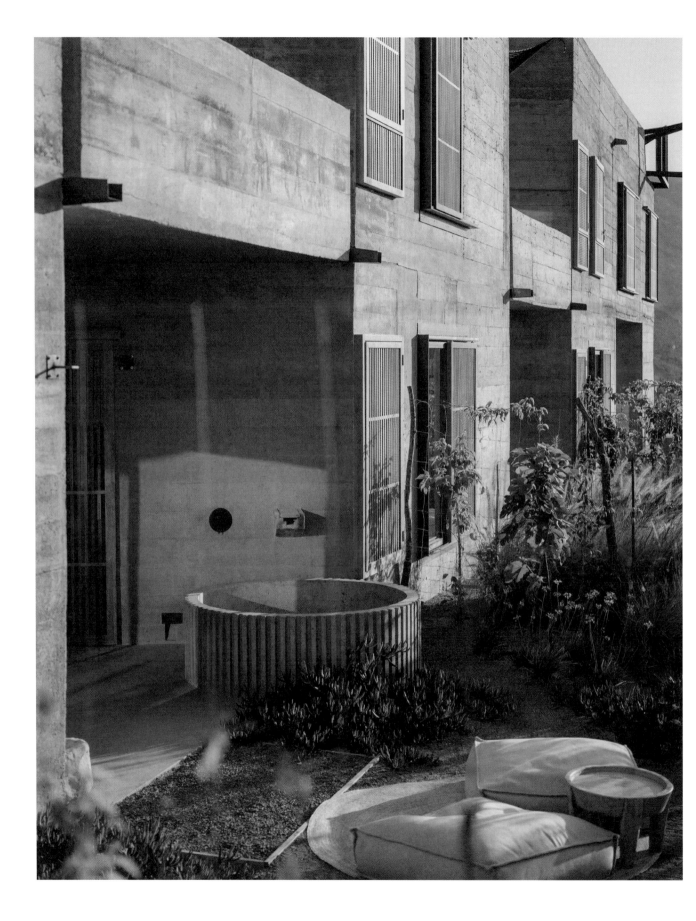

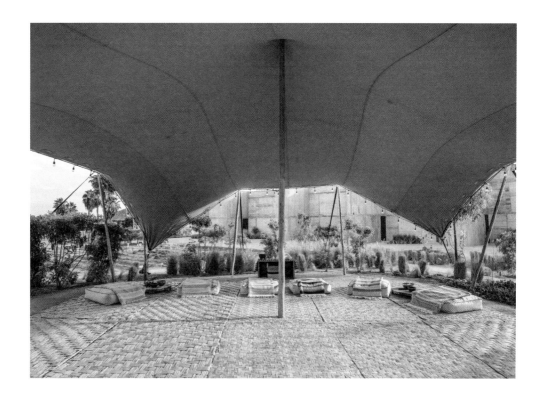

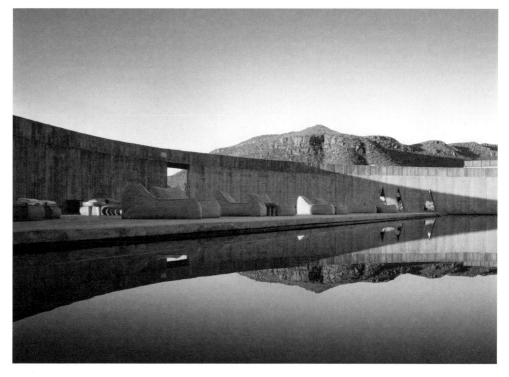

OPPOSITE One of the garden suites features a private garden, outdoor terrace, and soak tub. ABOVE Guests lounging around the half-moon pool have views of the mountains and Las Palmas Beach in the distance. At night this space becomes a popular gathering spot around a fire pit.

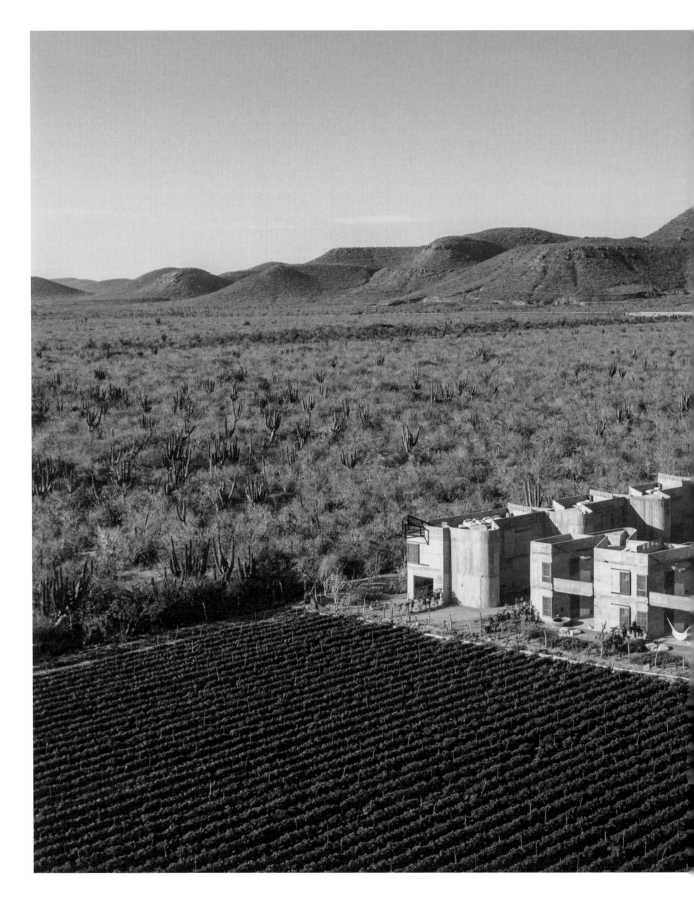

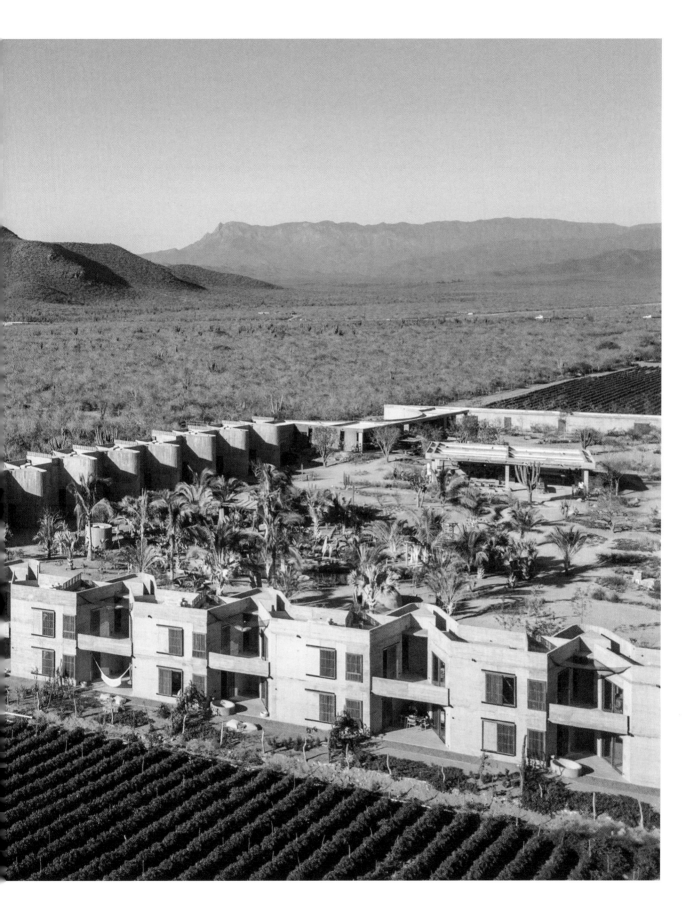

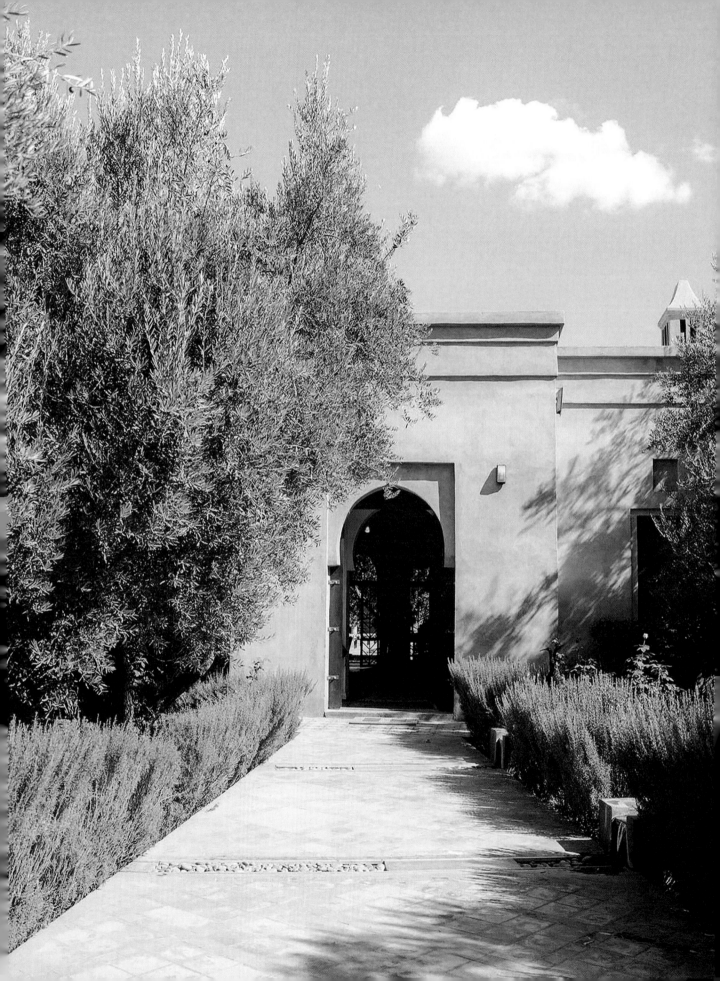

LUXURY CREATIVE AND HEALTH-CONSCIOUS RETREAT PACKAGES WITH A MOROCCAN VIBE

Peacock Pavilions
Marrakech, Morocco

Designed to promote WELL-BEING AND FUN, this luxury boutique hotel boasts a swimming pool, an outdoor gym, an open-air cinema, and a yoga pavilion among its facilities.

Located in a private olive grove 10 miles (15 km) outside Marrakech, the Peacock Pavilions' 8.5-acre (3.5-hectare) estate boasts three pavilions, two luxury bungalows, and breathtaking views of the Atlas Mountains. Designed and built—and lived in—by American designer and author Maryam Montague and her husband Chris Redecke, Peacock Pavilions is run as a "give-back" boutique hotel, which also supports a local non-profit organization called Project Soar. Its aim is to empower local teenage girls through arts and sports alongside health and English language education.

The hotel's primary communal spaces can be found in and around the Main Pavilion, which is surrounded by hundreds of fragrant rose bushes. Beyond a grand, domed reception area is an African-inspired indoor dining salon with an arcaded outdoor terrace lined with tile-topped tables. There is also a small library of books and a boutique called the Souk by M. Montague, where guests can buy products from the owner's Tribal Chic range of home accessories, fashion, and textiles.

Lodging for up to 16 people is spread among the other buildings. The Atlas Pavilion, draped in bougainvillea, has three en suite bedrooms, a spacious shared living room, and private rooftop terraces overlooking the estate. The Medina Pavilion has three en suite bedrooms, a shared living room, a dining room, a fully equipped kitchen, and a private rose garden. The two Dawn and Dusk bungalows each sleep two and have an en suite bathroom and private lounge. Guests are welcome to rent out the entire property,

OPPOSITE The approach to the hotel is lined with olive trees and lavender. The terracotta facade of the building takes cues from Moorish architecture.

a pavilion, or an individual room depending on their group size. Meals are served in several locations; dining areas change according to the weather and the number of people. They include an arcaded terrace, the pool cabana, and a unique painted Arabian dining tent. Menus feature farm-to-table, authentic Moroccan cuisine and a fixed daily menu that relies on local, fresh ingredients, some from the estate's own gardens. Dinner at the hotel includes three delicious courses and ends with a herbal tea.

Through the year, the hotel runs a program of seven-day retreats focused on yoga, meditation, arts, crafts, and Moroccan culture. The Private Insider Retreat, led by the hotel's owner, includes a guided tour of Marrakech's *medina*, a luxury pampering spa experience, high tea at the lavish Royal Mansour hotel, a visit to the Majorelle Gardens, and a nomad-inspired camel ride, among other activities. ✳

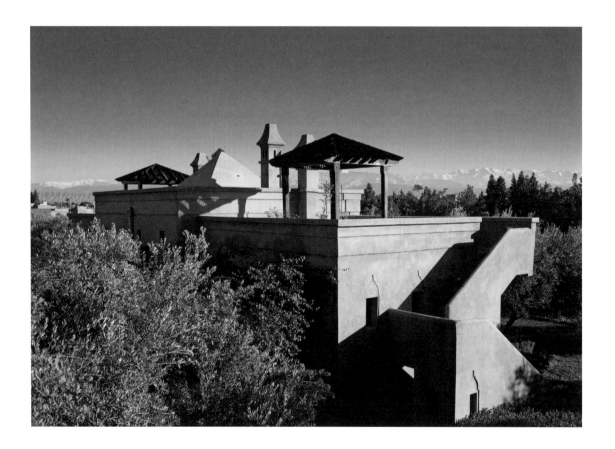

ABOVE The main hotel building seen from the rear, with the Atlas mountains in the distance. OPPOSITE The elegant reception hall shows paper lanterns suspended from the domed ceiling and hand-knotted rugs on the tiled floor.

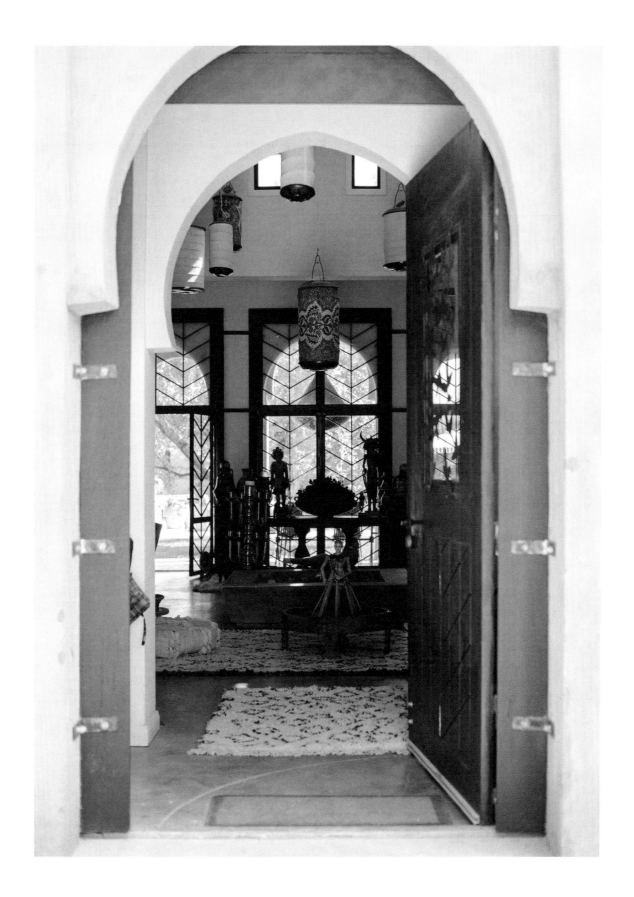

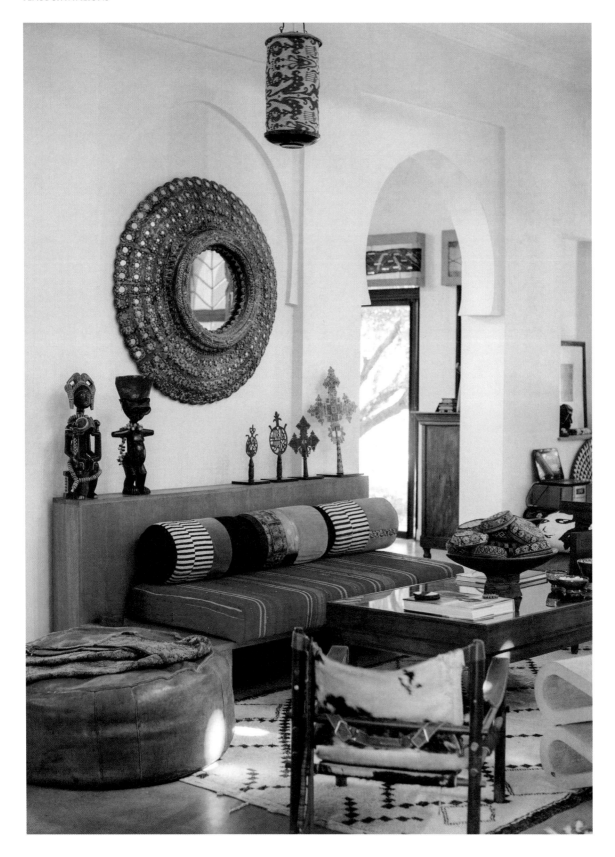

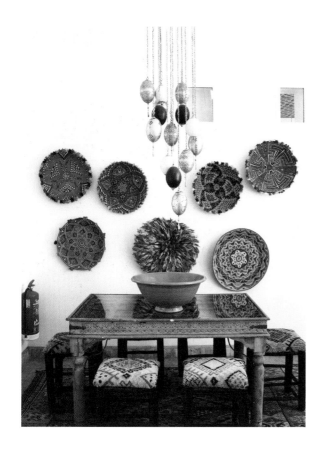

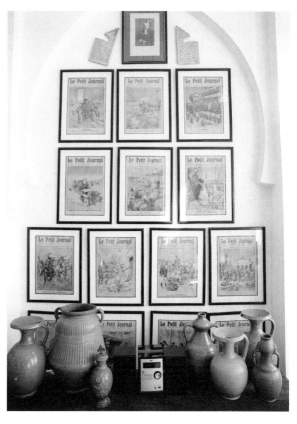

OPPOSITE AND ABOVE The owners are passionate about Moroccan design and all the rooms were styled using local, handmade decorative items and hand-dyed textiles and soft furnishings. In the boutique souk at the hotel guests can buy similar wares.

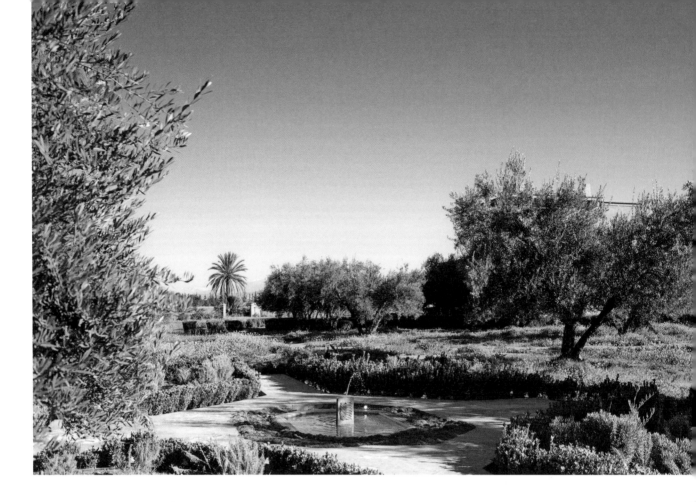

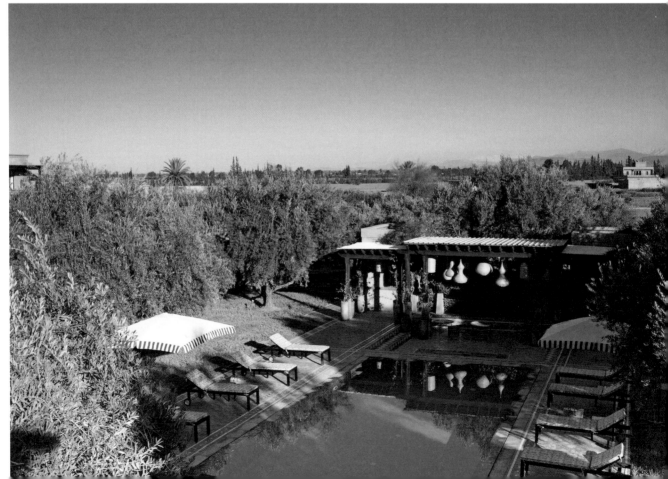

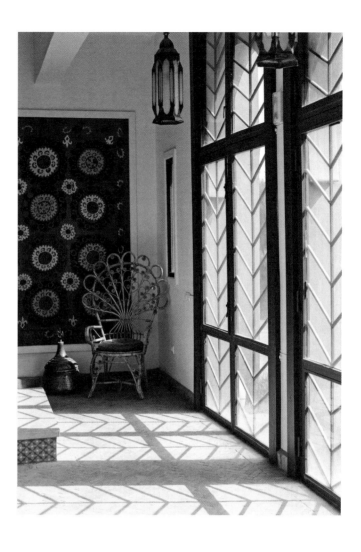

OPPOSITE The hotel is surrounded by well-kept gardens and tranquil spaces for guests to relax in. Among the various facilities on the grounds are a communal swimming pool, an outdoor gym, an outdoor cinema, a yoga pavilion, and a painted dining tent.

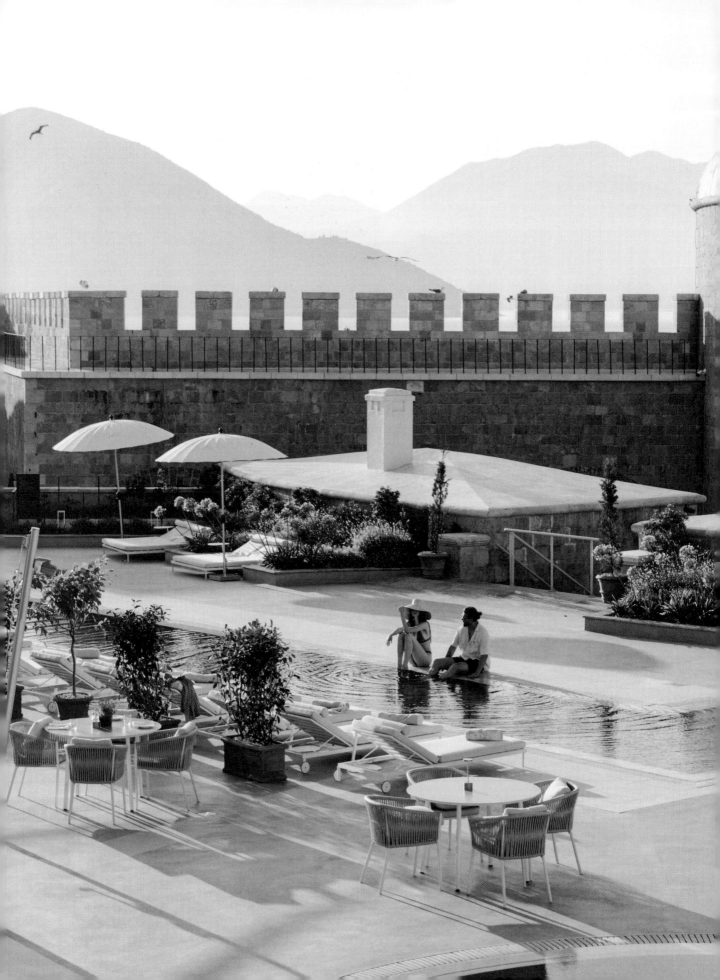

A HARMONIOUS BLEND OF RELAXATION AND ENRICHMENT IN THE ADRIATIC SEA

Mamula Island Hotel
Herceg Novi, Montenegro

With a HOLISTIC APPROACH to its guests' well-being, this island resort blends traditional with modern practices to ensure that every wellness journey is as INNOVATIVE as it is REVITALIZING.

Mamula Island is the site of a beautifully restored 19th-century fortress in the Bay of Kotor, Montenegro. The whole of this fortress resort is dedicated to well-being, with 32 guest rooms and a holistic spa with a glass-covered courtyard. Guests can dine at any one of three restaurants and have unlimited access to three outdoor swimming pools and a private beach. The resort is the ideal location for an immersive experience of rejuvenation and relaxation surrounded by little more than sky and sea.

With its spa services, cultural programming, and culinary expertise, the Mamula Island Hotel guarantees guests a multifaceted experience deeply rooted in the locale and its heritage. During their stay, they can unwind and soak in the idyllic surroundings, indulge in fine-dining, enjoy operatic arias in the atrium, and take part in hands-on creative experiences through the hotel's Artist in Residence project.

On the ground floor of the fortress's main tower at the heart of the resort, the Mamula Spa offers a range of exclusive therapies that use organic skincare products inspired by the island's natural beauty and resources. Treatments are based on natural materials, such as local limestone and Adriatic Sea sponges, and are designed to activate the body's nervous system for profound and lasting results. Among the facilities in the spa are Finnish and herbal saunas, a steam bath, relaxation areas, two private treatment rooms, and an aqua flotation zone. Guests can book in for a range of holistic therapies that include sound healing, meditation and energy clearing, and movement sessions such

OPPOSITE Guests relax on the pool deck, dipping their toes in the water. This is a popular gathering spot for drinks and all-day dining.

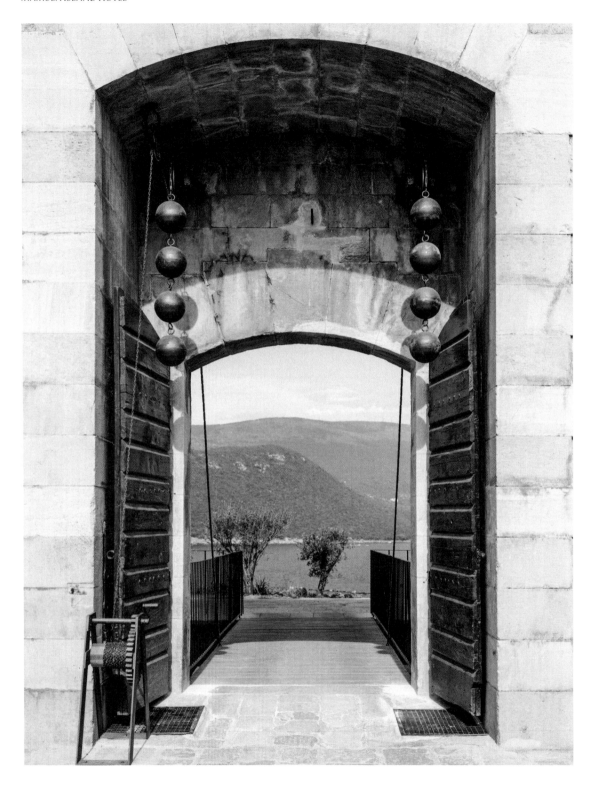

ABOVE On arrival to the island by speedboat, guests find themselves in front of an imposing arched gateway with a wooden drawbridge. Across the bridge is a large, welcoming, stone-paved courtyard with views to the sea. OPPOSITE Simple, comfortable indoor and outdoor spaces for yoga and relaxation.

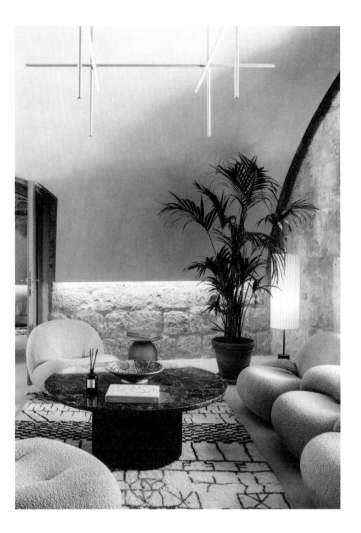

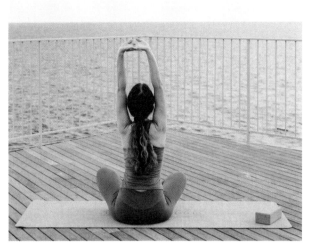

as yoga, Pilates, and breathwork. The hotel's 32 guest rooms and suites are divided in two collections: Heritage and New. The Heritage rooms—Sky Suites and Sea View Suites—can be found in the fort itself. Furnished with solid oak furniture and natural textiles, the rooms retain many of the fort's original features, including curved stone walls and picture-framed windows that once housed military cannons. The New rooms include eight Adriatic Balcony rooms with a shared garden to the front and private terraces to the rear. With floor-to-ceiling windows, they are light and bright and have stunning views. Additional amenities in some of the pricier suites include a private Jacuzzi, a sauna, a two-seat cinema, and a telescope for star-gazing. All of the rooms have a palette that draws on the surrounding landscape—natural, earthy tones mixed with bright colors.   ✳

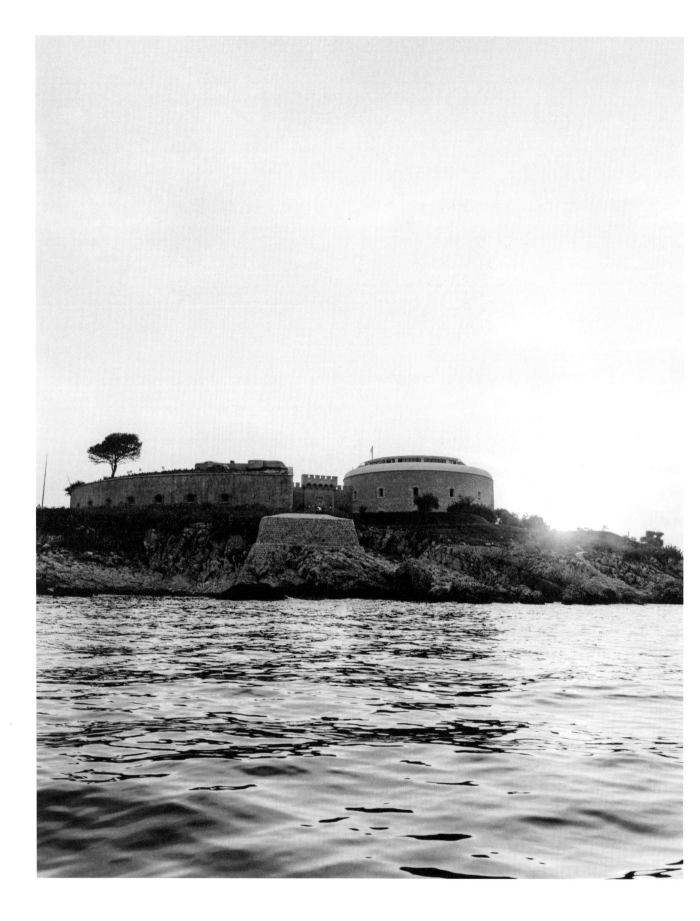

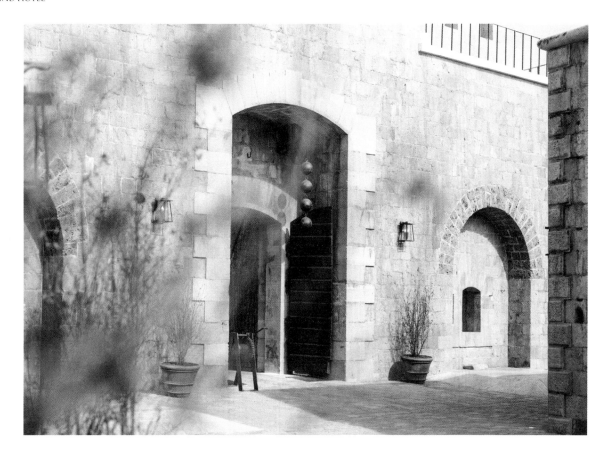

OPPOSITE Mamula Island is completely occupied by the hotel. The original fortress building was faithfully restored using local stone. Beyond the tower lies an internal courtyard with three pools and a bar-restaurant.

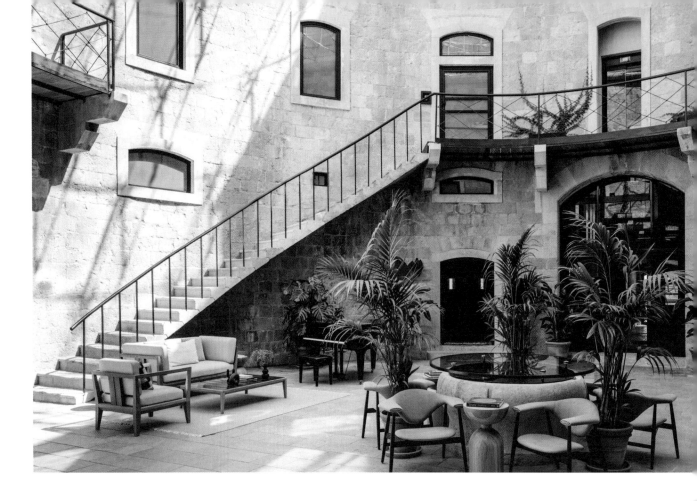

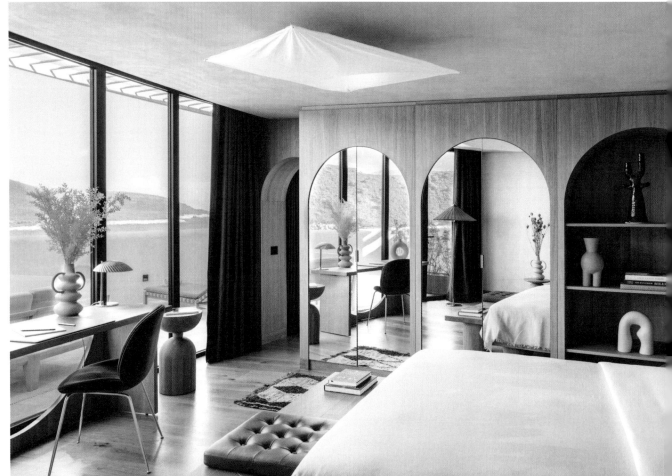

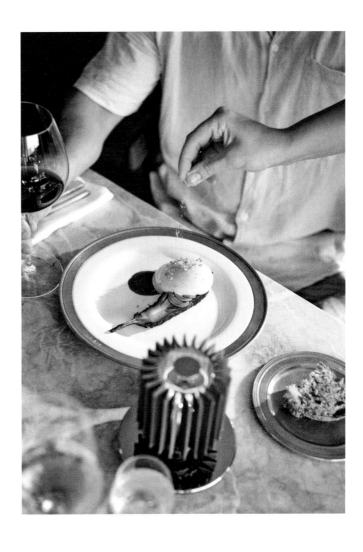

OPPOSITE, TOP This communal space at the center of the Spa Tower is often used to stage concerts.
OPPOSITE, BOTTOM The Panoramic Suite living rooms have floor-to-ceiling windows and a private terrace.
The palette draws from the island's landscape, with natural, earthy tones combined with soothing colors.

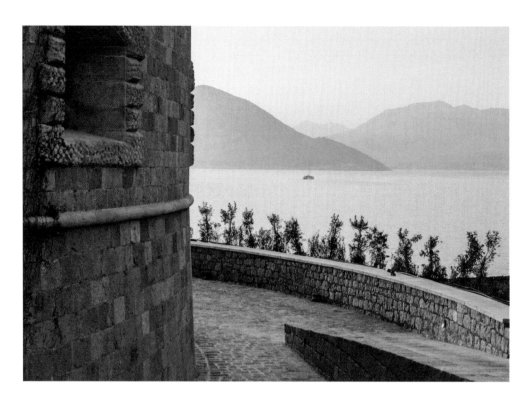

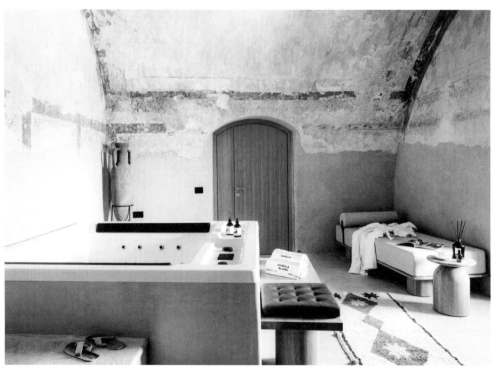

ABOVE AND OPPOSITE The Sky Suites are on the first floor of the Spa Tower. Many features of the original fort were retained, including the frescoes adorning the walls and ceilings, and the old stone walls keep the place cool in the summer.

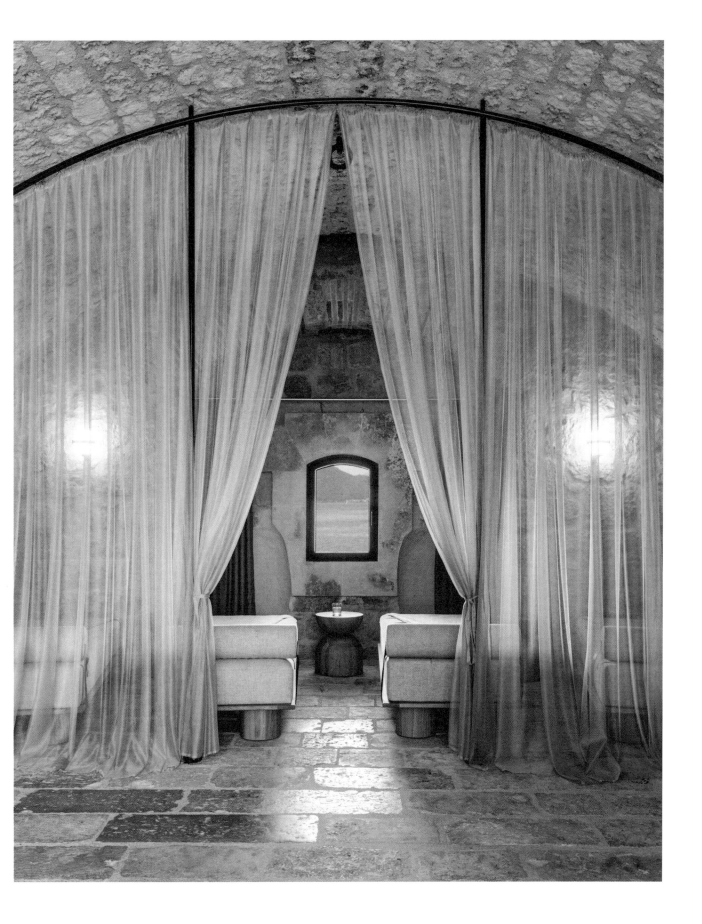

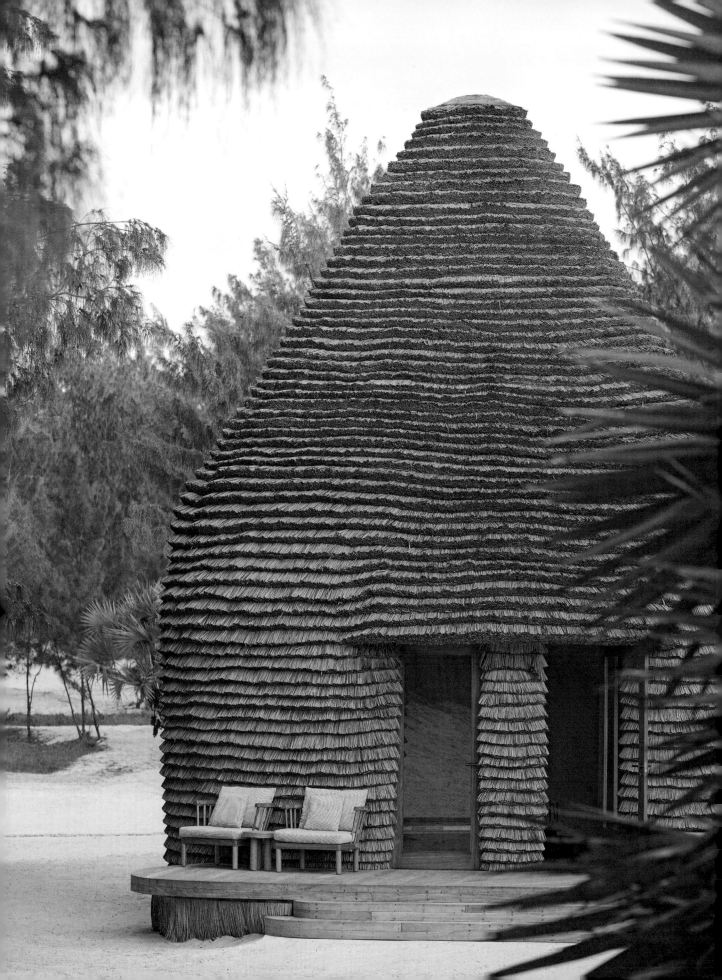

A CELEBRATION OF CULTURE, CRAFT, AND HERITAGE IN AN UNTOUCHED ISLAND SETTING

Kisawa Sanctuary

Benguerra Island, Mozambique

With 11 residences, each located within its own acre of beachfront and forest, Kisawa is Africa's first permanent OCEAN OBSERVATORY *and the world's first property to open in tandem with its own marine research center.*

Kisawa Sanctuary is home to some of the richest yet least explored subtropical ecosystems in the Indian Ocean and occupies 740 acres (300 hectares) of beachfront on Benguerra Island, Mozambique. More than 150 bird species from flamingos to parrots call this island home, as do the rare dugong and samango monkey. The island's abundant marine life includes humpback whales, sea turtles, marlin, tuna, and dolphins.

Set against this idyllic backdrop are 11 luxury residences occupying their own secluded patches of unspoiled terrain. There is a single bungalow for two or several bungalows grouped for larger parties, located either on the cove side of the island or sheltered among the sand dunes along the island's ocean side. Each residence has a shaded day area with an outdoor kitchen and a pantry stocked to its guests' preferences and a private swimming pool. Interiors celebrate Africa's rich cultural history, furnished sympathetically with unique art and antiques sourced from across the continent alongside locally made bespoke furniture. Colorful patterns and prints are evocative of the region, ensuring a thoughtful and authentic sense of place.

At the heart of Kisawa Sanctuary are several shared spaces dedicated to dining, relaxation, and well-being. The resort's four restaurants have menus focusing on seasonal, organic ingredients grown or produced locally. And among the sand dunes, the Natural Wellness Center offers guests individual treatments or personalized programs rooted in Ayurvedic medicine, including a state-of-the-art Japanese Iyashi Dome sauna that utilizes gentle infrared heat to promote healing.

OPPOSITE Dubbed the "yoga nest," this domed structure is dedicated to yoga and Pilates sessions. The Natural Wellness Center and a fully equipped gym are also nearby.

BELOW AND RIGHT Guests are welcome to book in for all manner of treatments and massages in the Natural Wellness Center or in the privacy of their own rooms. OPPOSITE The interiors boast antiques alongside locally made bespoke furniture.

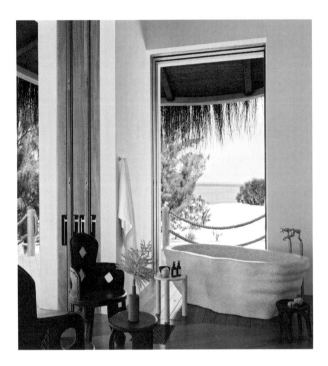

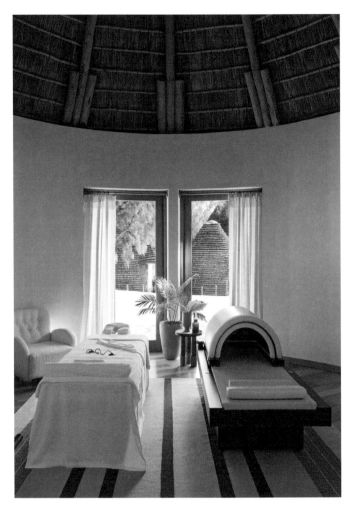

With a minimum stay of three nights, visitors are invited to make use of an incredible range of activities designed for luxury relaxation and recuperation. These include a 24-hour jet-lag recovery treatment with a 60-minute massage, water sports such as sea kayaking, paddle boarding, and snorkeling, and tailor-made excursions and explorations around the island. In addition, each residence has the use of a colorful electric beach buggy for getting around the place. The Kisawa Sanctuary was founded by entrepreneur and philanthropist Nina Flohr, whose work seeks to combine luxury hospitality with environmental conservation. On Benguerra Island, this is achieved by pairing the for-profit sanctuary with the Bazaruto Center for Scientific Studies, a nonprofit organization dedicated to marine science and research. ✳

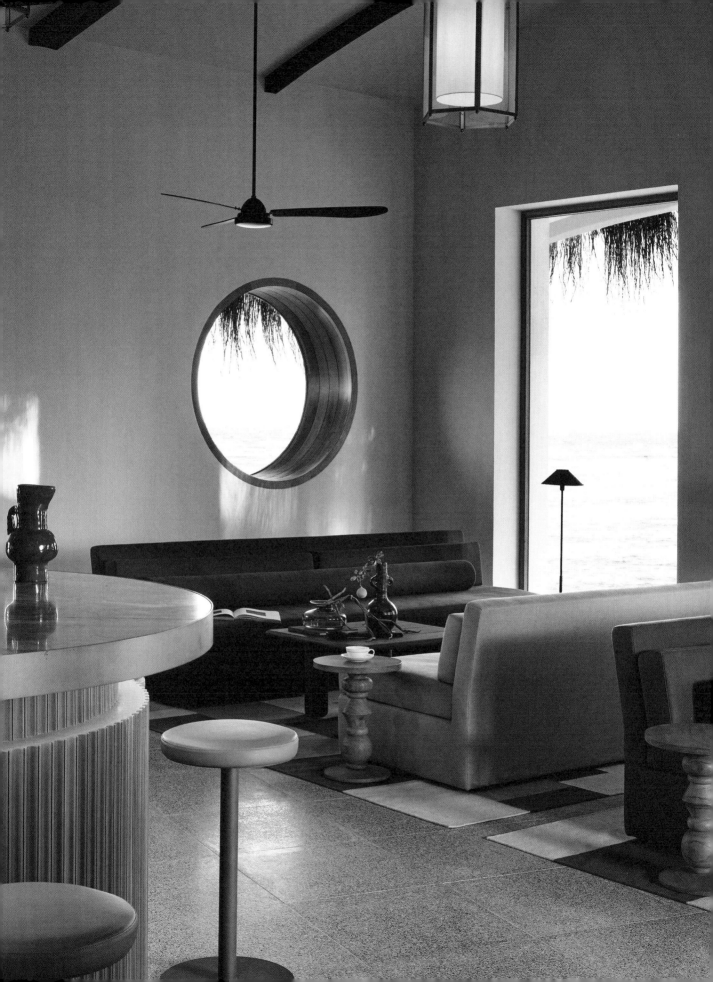

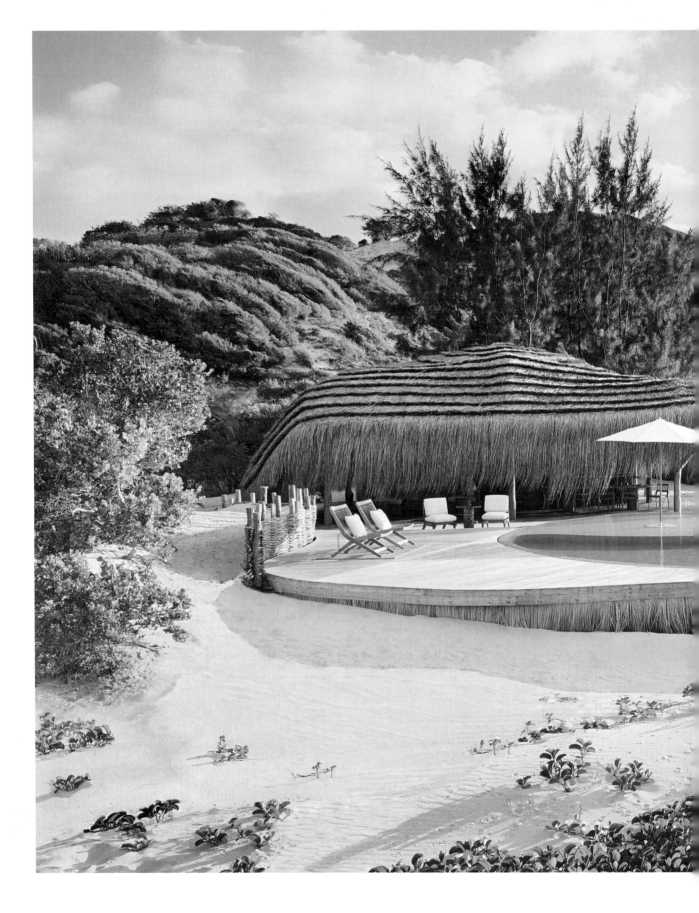

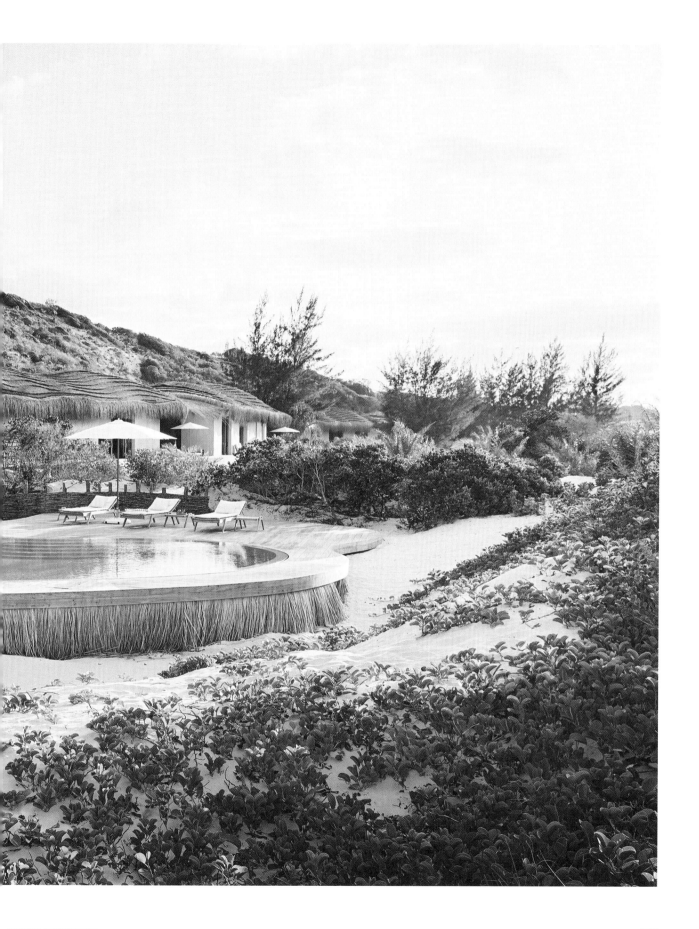

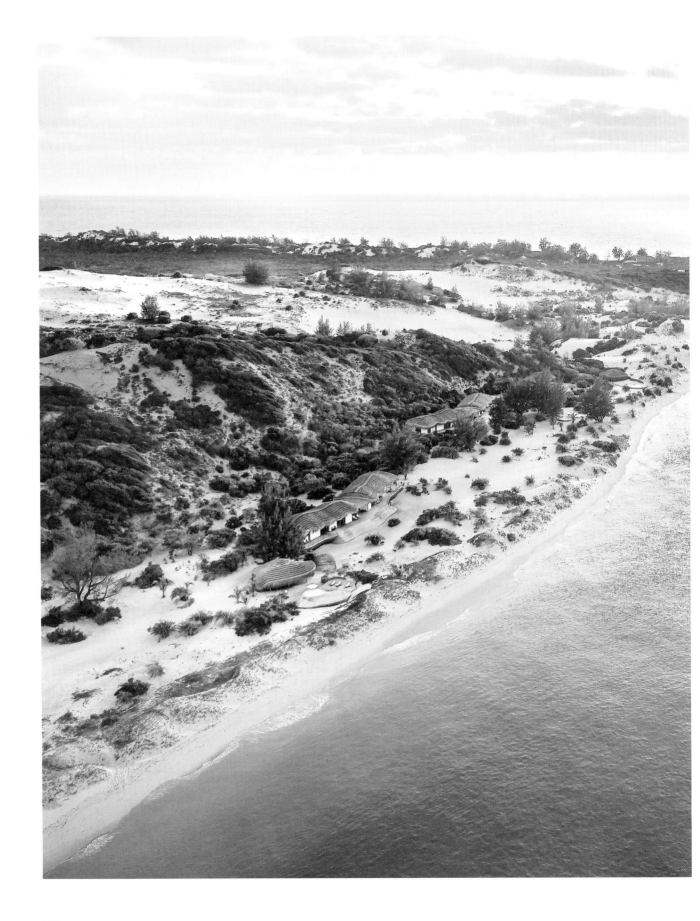

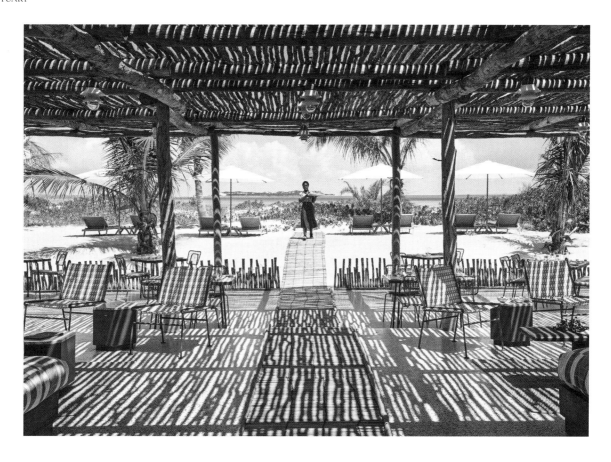

ABOVE The Cove Mussassa offers one of several dining experiences at this beach resort—a well-shaded, relaxed beach cafe that is open pretty much all day and well into the evening. The menu focuses on fresh seafood and Mediterranean-style sharing plates.

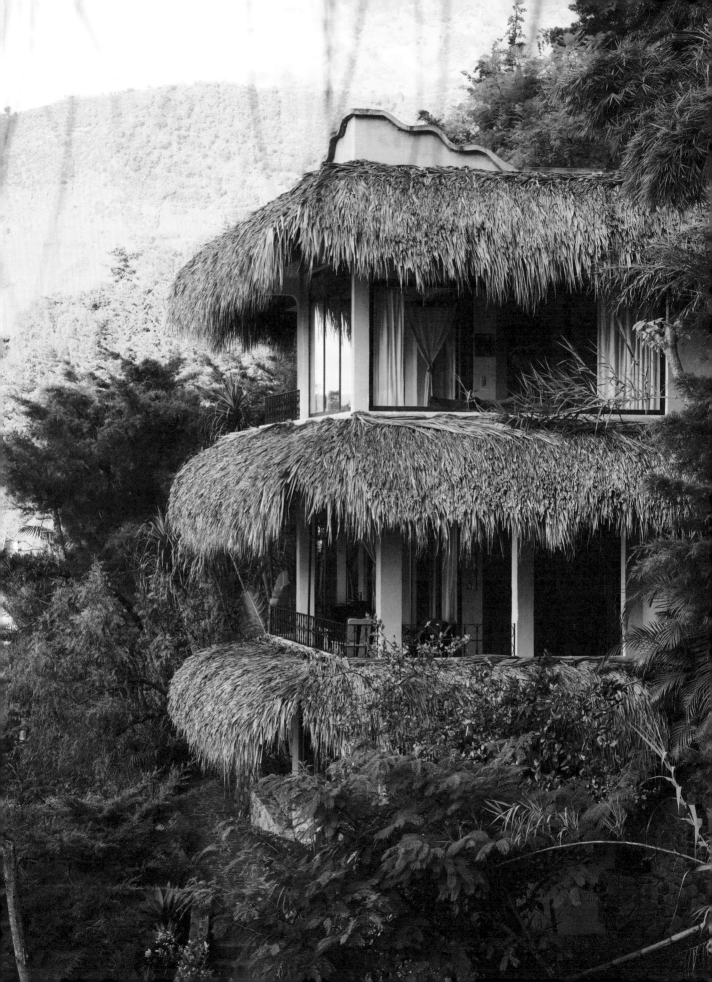

A CENTER FOR HOLISTIC HEALING IN THE HEART OF THE GUATEMALAN HIGHLANDS

Villa Sumaya

Santa Cruz la Laguna, Guatemala

With a wide range of outdoor activities and personalized wellness treatments—and accessible only by boat— this is the PERFECT PLACE in which to UNWIND and RECHARGE in the most tranquil of surroundings.

The Villa Sumaya retreat and wellness center is in Santa Cruz la Laguna, a traditional Mayan village nestled on the slopes of the Sierra Madre mountain range, which rises above Lake Atitlán in Guatemala. Stunning all year round, the region has two primary seasons: dry and rainy. Typically running from November to April, the dry season is the resort's busiest as it brings little rainfall. Things are quieter in May through June and September through October, when the weather is less predictable and seasonal storms can last for days. However, this is also when the landscape is particularly beautiful, lush, and green.

The center comprises a number of buildings lining the shores of the lake and set within beautifully landscaped gardens. Of its 22 guestrooms, the most luxurious are the Ginger Suites, each with views across the lake, a private balcony, elegant antique furnishings, and modern bathrooms. The Lotus House rooms are spacious, with private baths, balconies, and stunning views while the Maya Rose House rooms have semi-private patio spaces with cozy seating. Higher up, three Skyline Bungalows perch on the hillside among the trees and feature queen beds, unique bathrooms, and magnificent views of the lake.

Public spaces include two large studios, two open-air platforms, two solar-powered hot pools and saunas, a year-round swimming pool, and several lounges. During a stay at Villa Sumaya, guests will also find hammocks and countless relaxation spaces dotted around the gardens for moments of quiet contemplation.

OPPOSITE Characteristic of the local vernacular architecture, the buildings at this retreat have bushy thatches on each floor to shield the rooms within from the midday heat.

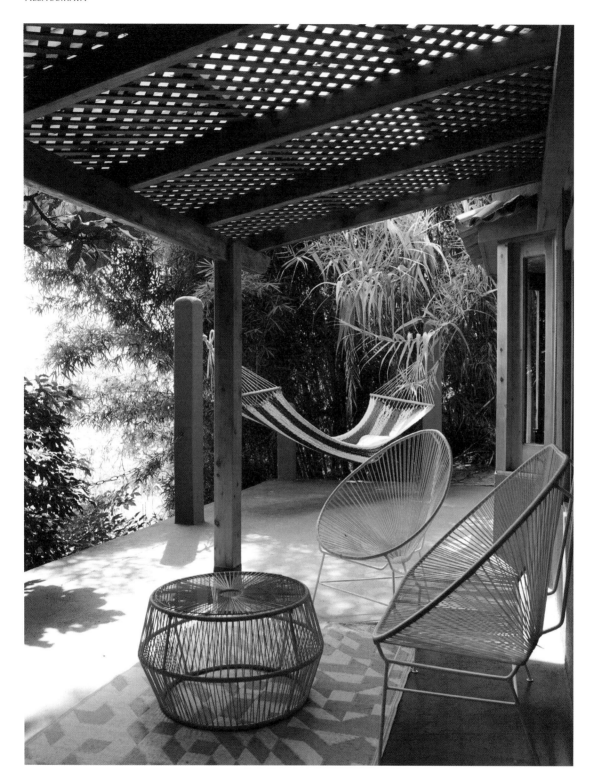

ABOVE Many rooms, like the Lotus Suite, have generous, partially shaded terraces with stunning views across the lake.
OPPOSITE, RIGHT All of the colors here are warm and inviting. Guest rooms are decorated in earthy tones, frequently married with sumptuous red, blue, and purple textiles.

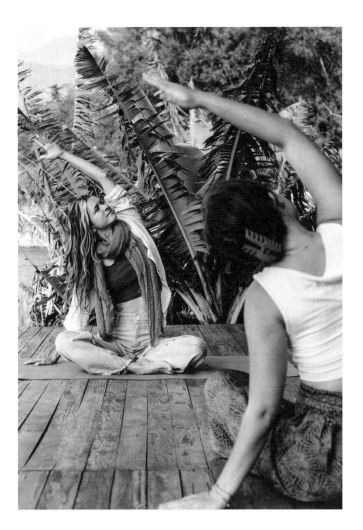

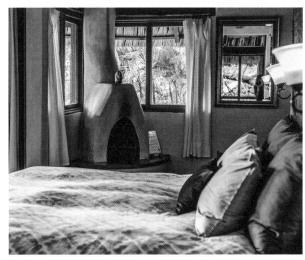

Guests have access to the on-site Harmony Spa, which offers customized sessions with skilled practitioners. Depending on the season and availability, treatments might include Swedish neuro-lumbar massage, Thai massage, *Reiki,* reflexology, energy therapy, acupuncture, Ayurvedic massage, shiatsu massage, deep tissue massage, and facial treatments. Those looking for spiritual healing can also book in for astrology readings in both Western and Mayan traditions. The center also offers a 5* Personal Retreat Package—a seven-day course that might include the ritual of the sacred sweat lodge and a Mayan fire ceremony, with daily yoga or intuitive art sessions.

A retreat at the center includes full board at the on-site restaurant, where meals center on freshly prepared homemade buffets based on a vegetarian diet accompanied by fresh breads and homemade tortillas.   *

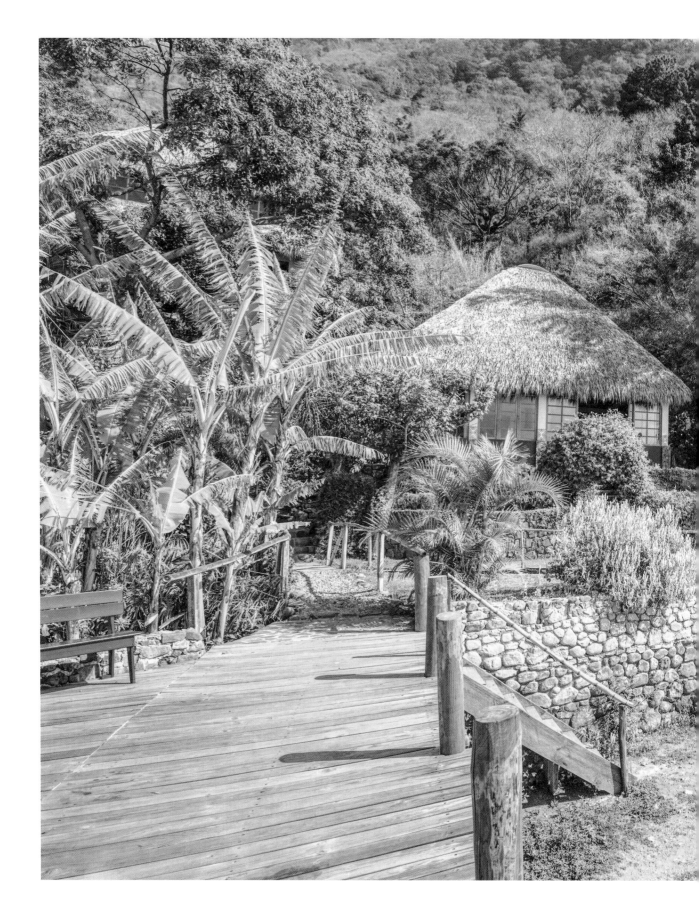

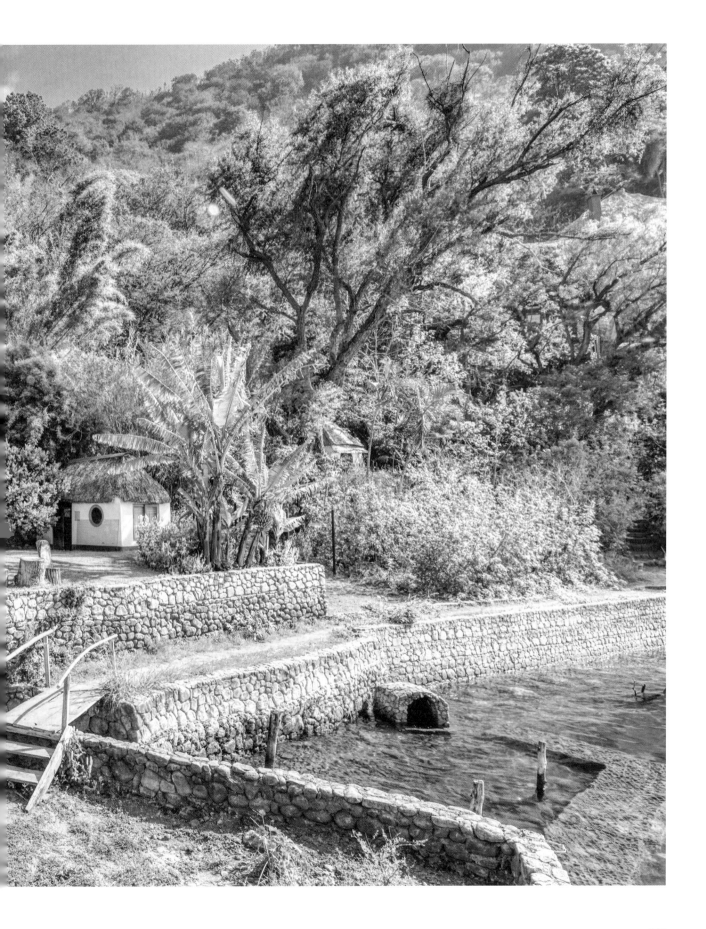

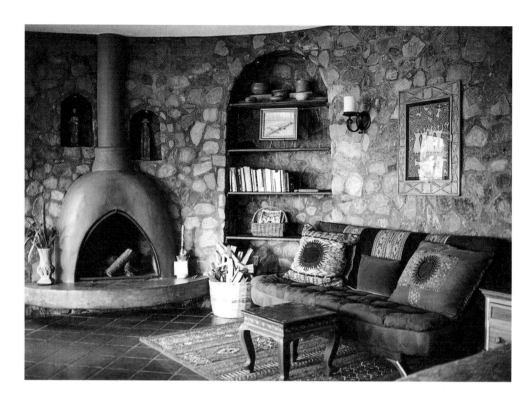

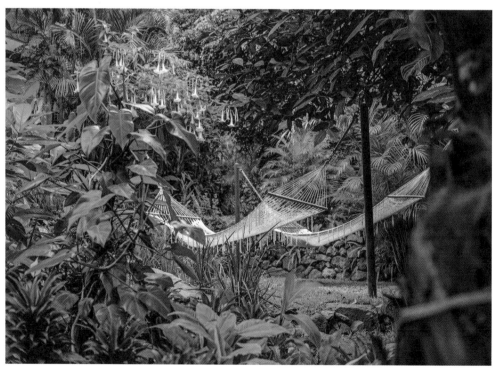

ABOVE Inside and out guests find all manner of inviting spaces in which to relax, whether in a cozy salon with a log-burning stove or in hammocks suspended from trees. OPPOSITE The Ganesh Healing Hut is one of four spaces in which guests can indulge in a wide variety of spa services.

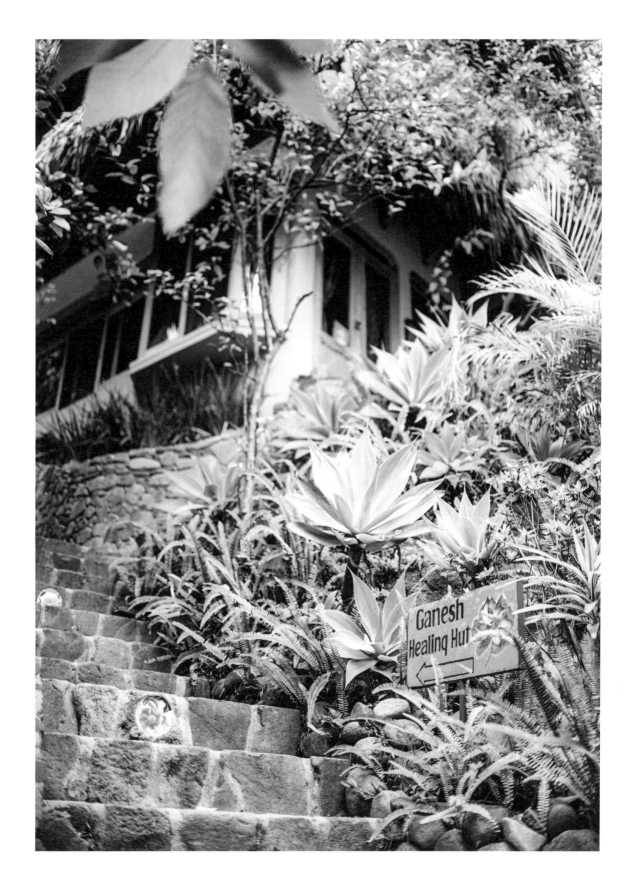

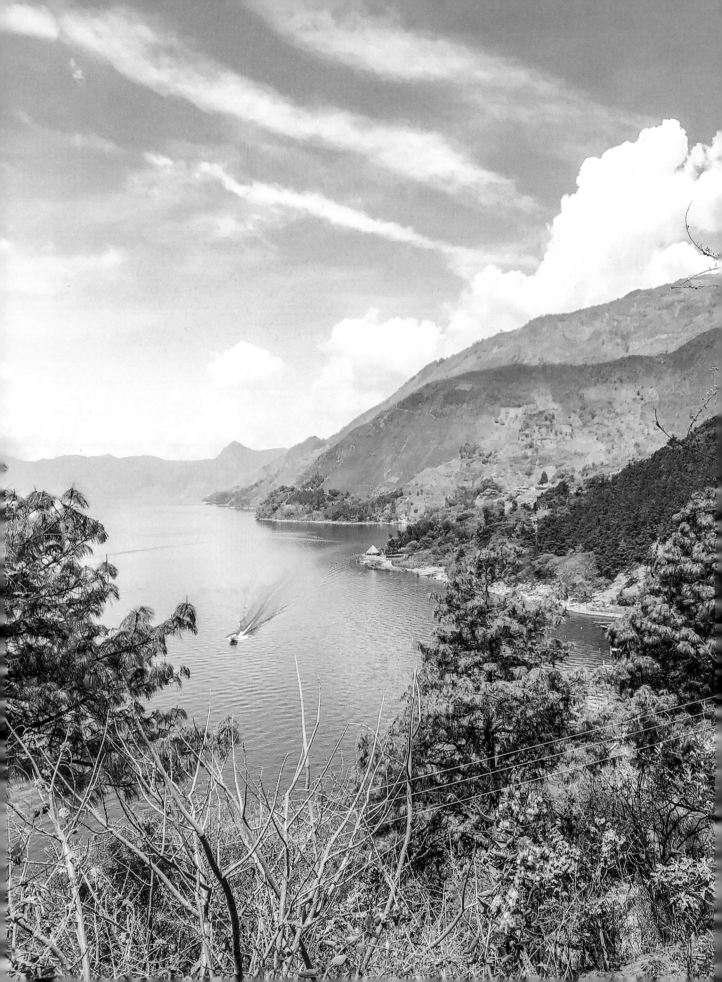

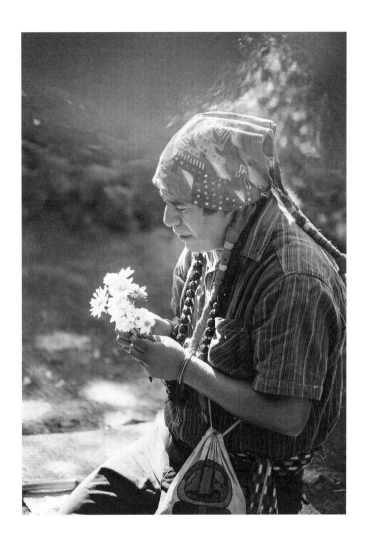

ABOVE A shaman performs a fire ceremony. Mayan in tradition, it involves creating beautiful offerings that are then consumed by the fire, invoking awareness and connection with all that is. It serves as a reminder for us to leave behind our busy minds and conditioned concept of self.

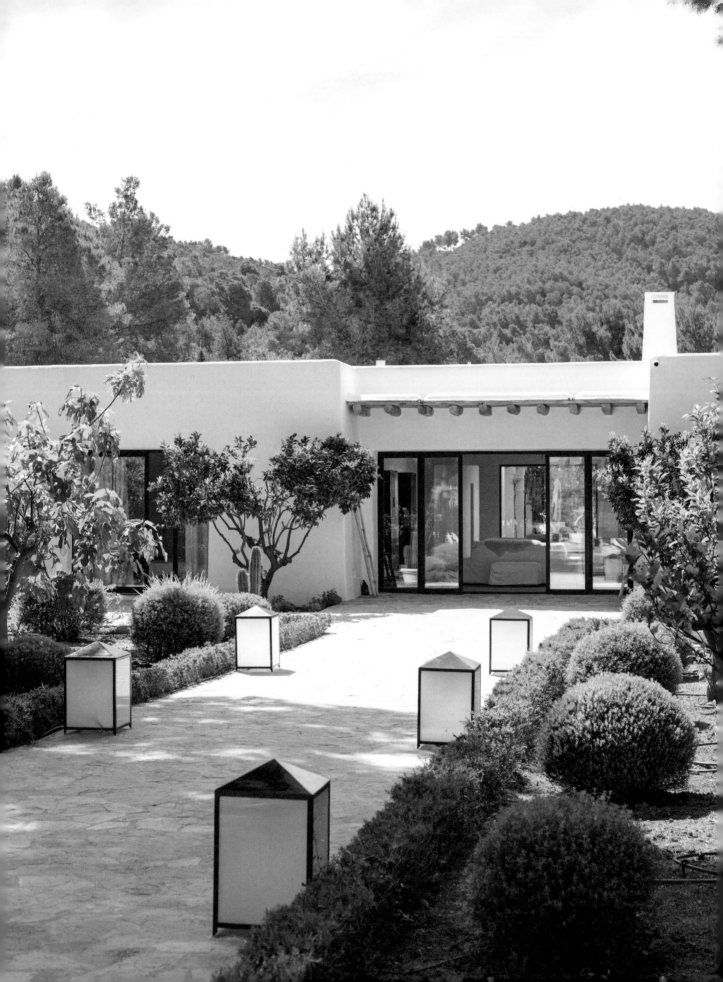

Wylder Ibiza
San Miguel, Ibiza, Spain

A FIVE-DAY WELLNESS AND CULTURAL RETREAT ON THE SPANISH ISLAND OF IBIZA

This island resort offers guests a taste of the local culture and natural beauty while taking part in a wide range of MINDFUL PRACTICES and outdoor adventures.

Guests arriving at Wylder Ibiza can look forward to a unique wellness experience that has been carefully designed by host Charlotte Townend. A qualified yoga teacher, Townend teams up with local instructors, restaurants, and therapists to offer guests a five-day program that combines yoga with mindful practices, outdoor adventures, and unique workshops.

Scheduled during spring (April/May) and fall (September/October), the retreats are hosted at Can Terra, a beautiful villa in the sleepy Ibizan village of San Miguel. Townend herself offers a daily yoga session on a platform situated in a pine forest behind the house, overlooking the Mediterranean Sea. Additional health-focused activities include two Pilates sessions given by a local instructor, an evening breathwork session with a local practitioner, and a hike with the Other Face, a leading Ibiza-based hiking guide.

The villa has accommodation for up to 12 people in single or double-occupancy rooms. The rooms are light and bright, with whitewashed walls and simple furnishings, natural textiles, and stunning views out to sea. There is a communal swimming pool and guests gather to eat meals together around a large dining table on the terrace.

Wylder frequently collaborates with local restaurants for pop-ups during the retreats. Guests might find themselves tucking into Mexican street food at the local restaurant Chidas or taking part in an immersive cooking experience on the local farm Terra Viva. There, guests can meet the farmers, enjoy a tour of the farm, learn about their work on regeneration and permacultures, and cook a lunch using vegetables they have harvested

OPPOSITE Guests approach the luxury villa Can Terra through landscaped Mediterranean gardens. The building has a simple geometric structure and is whitewashed inside and out.

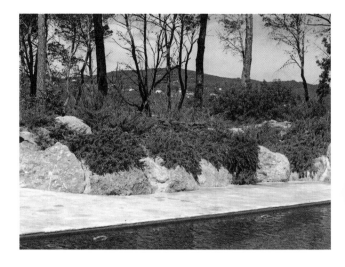

for themselves. Back at the retreat, nutritious plant-based dishes and freshly made juices and smoothies are prepared by the villa chef, Valentina.

All activities and meals on the retreat are included in the package, as is a fun jewelry-making workshop with local artisan Sylvie, an open-air movie night at the villa hosted by Cinema Paradiso Ibiza, and transfer to and from the airport. For an extra cost, guests can also enjoy a range of therapeutic beauty and body treatments administered by renowned local therapists. ✳

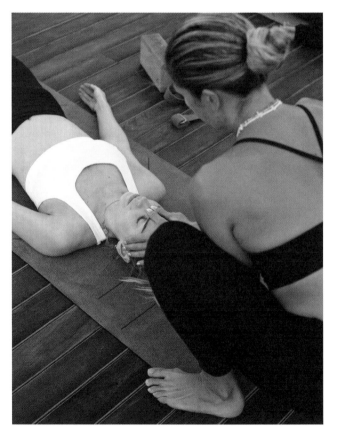

ABOVE AND OPPOSITE A teacher leads a class on the wooden yoga platform in the forest behind the villa—the warm air here is always fragrant with the smell of pine. The classes vary in style between energizing vinyasa and the slower, restorative yin yoga.

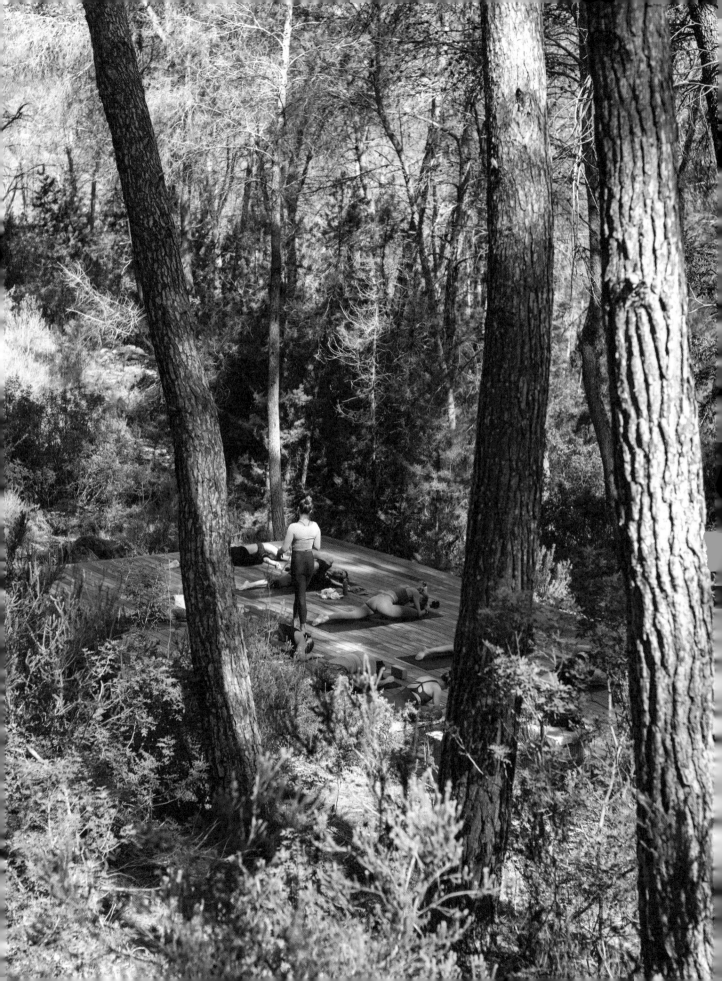

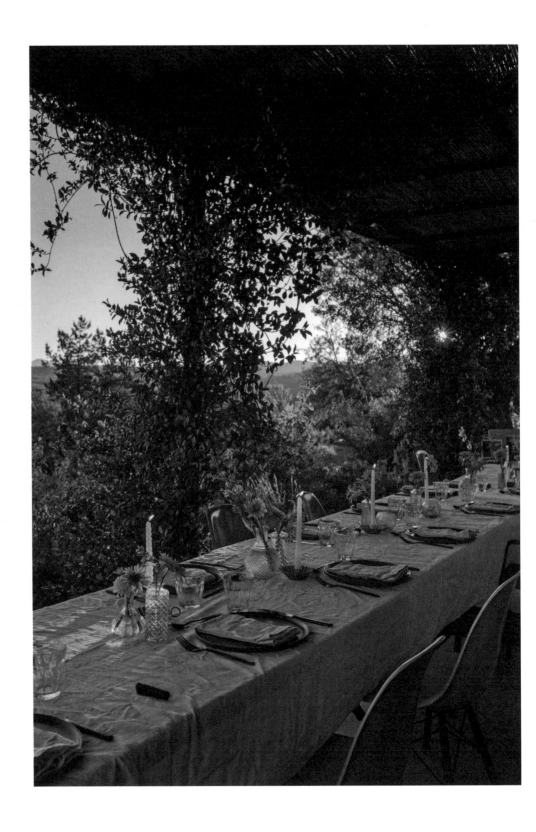

ABOVE With a menu focused on fresh, nutritious plant-based dishes, every meal served is a gastronomic delight. In the evenings, the guests eat together at sundown, sitting at a long, beautifully laid table in the most tranquil of natural surroundings.

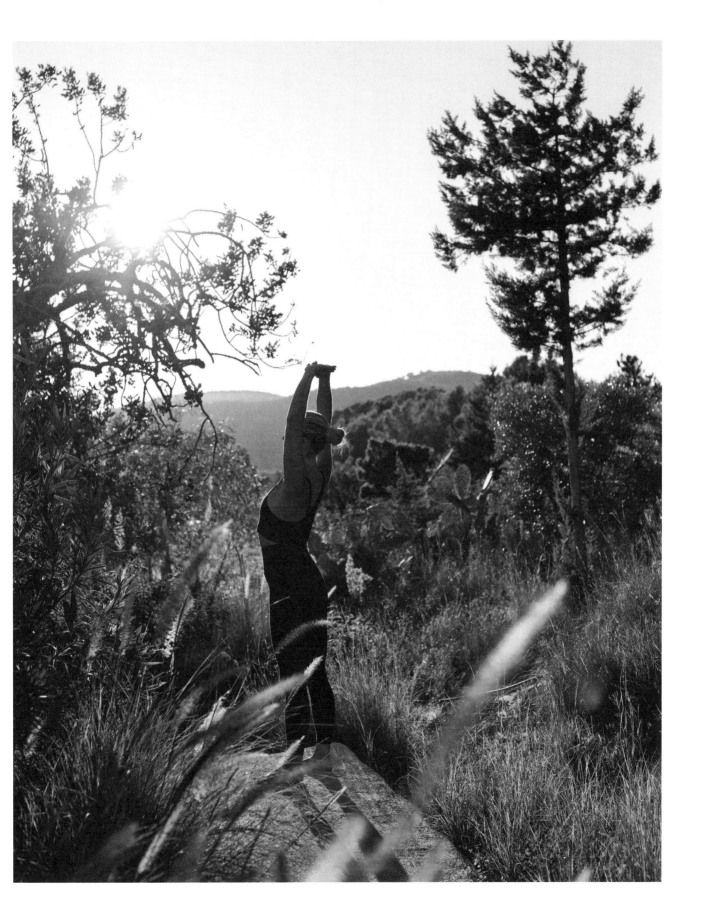

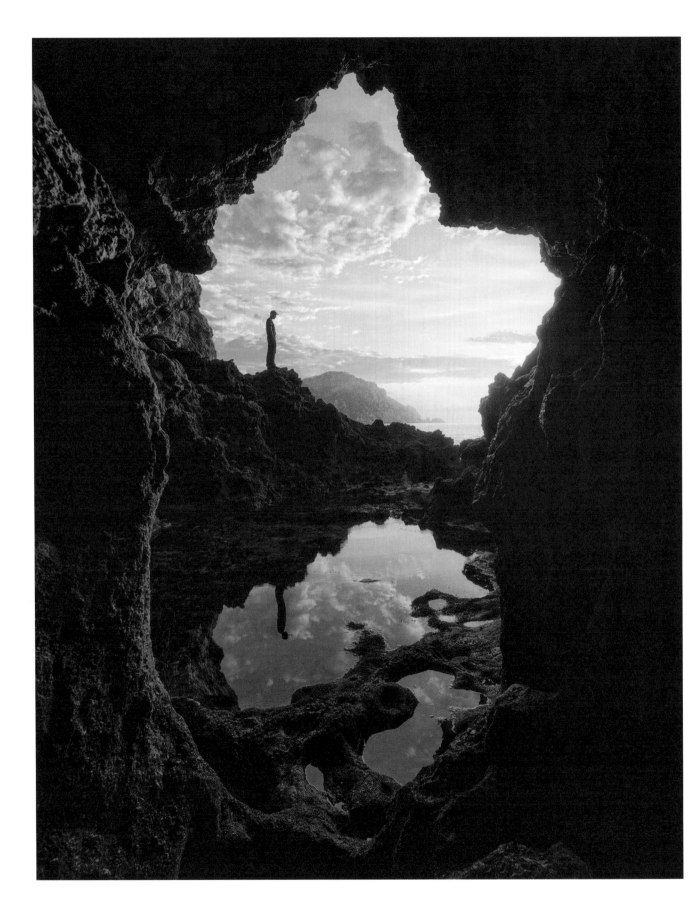

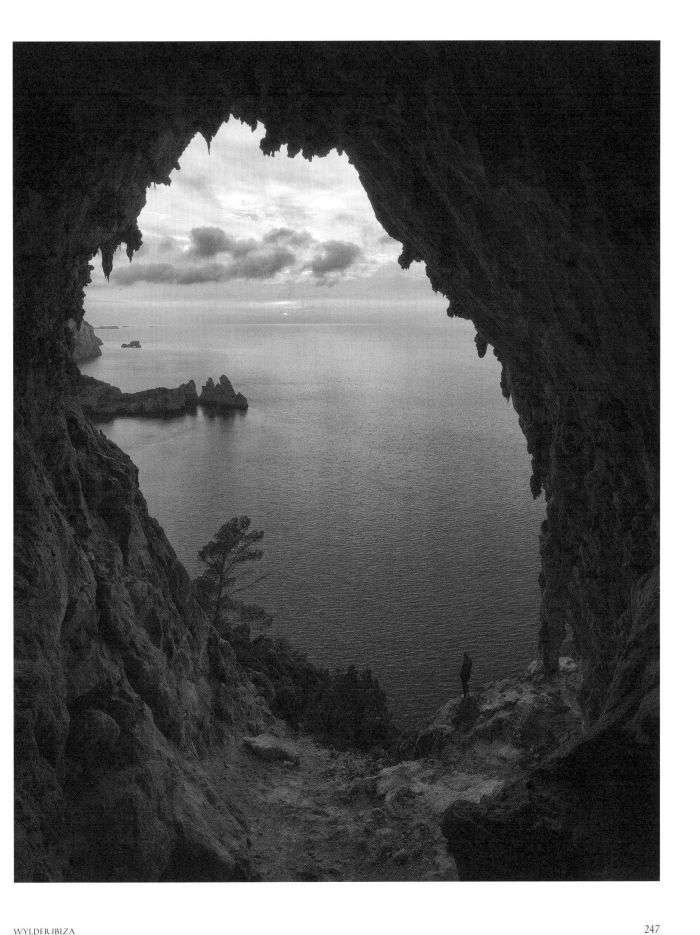

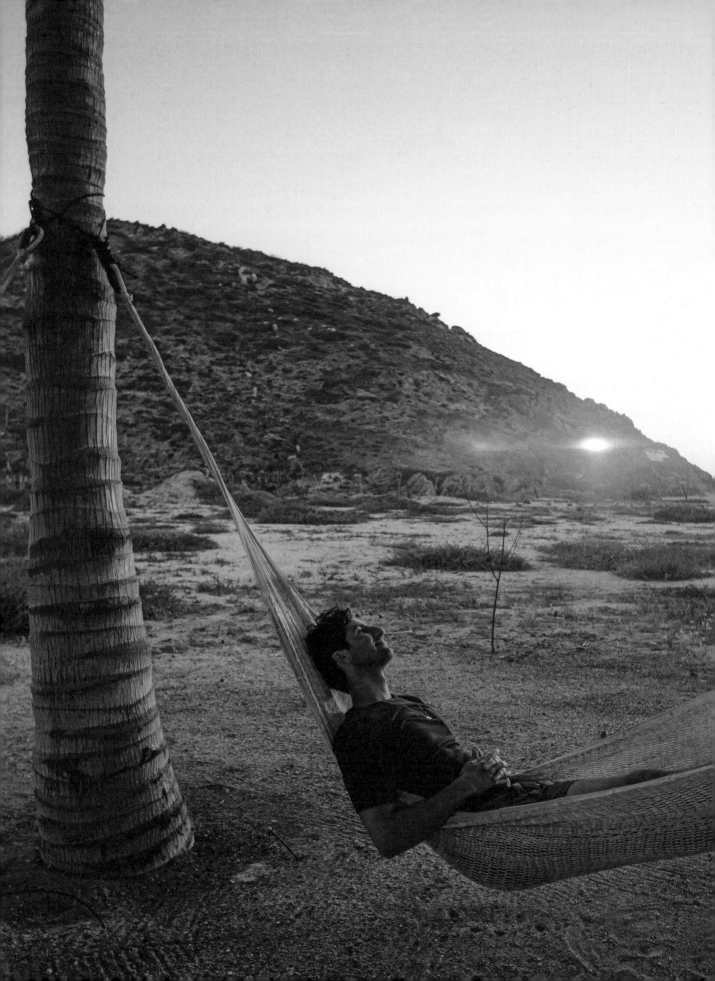

DAY-TO-DAY LIVING IN A YOGA COMMUNITY IN MEXICO'S STUNNING BAJA CALIFORNIA DESERT

Yandara Yoga Institute
Todos Santos, Mexico

In this magical resort where the DESERT MEETS THE SEA, *all-inclusive yoga retreats are specially designed to promote well-being—this is* OCEANFRONT GLAMPING *with a healthy twist.*

The Yandara Yoga Institute sits within 4 acres (1.6 hectares) of nature reserve in a stretch of the Baja California desert that flanks the Pacific Ocean in Mexico's Southern Baja Peninsula. With three yoga pavilions just a stone's throw from the beach, guests have phenomenal views of the Pacific Ocean and the Sierra de la Laguna mountain range. The stunning desert landscape that surrounds the resort is populated with plump aloe vera, blue agave, thick-stemmed trees, and majestic cacti. Functioning as both a teacher-training center and a yoga school, Yandara operates from mid-October to mid-July, when daytime temperatures average at a comfortable 70 °F (20 °C).

Retreats last anywhere from seven to 10 days at this secluded resort, and offer a program of wellness activities based on daily yoga and mediation sessions. Included in the price package are all meals, glamping-style accommodation, and a guided hike with stunning views. The retreats are themed and include a Winter Solstice Retreat, a Mindset Reset Retreat, and a Wild and Sacred Retreat. Additional services at the resort consist of astrology consultations, Reiki sessions, massage treatments, tea ceremonies, and sound baths.

While staying at Yandara, guests have three types of modest single- and double-occupancy accommodation to choose from: beachfront cabanas, eco-friendly cabins, and breathable canvas glamping tents. All have lights and electricity and are furnished with a contemporary rustic vibe; some even include en suite bathrooms. Meals at the resort are primarily vegetarian, with fresh local fish,

OPPOSITE Sunset is the perfect time for a hammock break—temperatures dip dramatically at night, but the air is still warm as the ground releases heat absorbed during the day.

eggs, and dairy products as optional extras. Papayas, bananas, oranges, and mangos grow in the resort's grounds as do most of the herbs and vegetables used in the recipes. Dishes are accompanied with homemade dressings and sauces, and there is always a well-stocked fruit bowl, an herbal tea station, and drinking water for refreshment throughout the day. Beside the three yoga pavilions, additional facilities at Yandara include a kitchen, communal dining and lounging areas, flush toilets, and showers. The retreat also has a saltwater pool for cooling down in the daytime and a firepit and hammocks for cozy gatherings at night, when temperatures can drop as low as 50 °F (10 °C) in the winter. Beyond the retreat, there are opportunities to explore the enchanting wonders of Todos Santos, just 15 minutes north by road.　＊

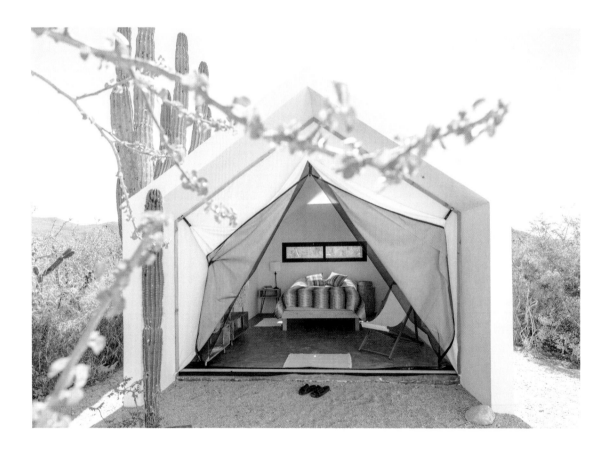

ABOVE The beachfront tents and cabanas are simply furnished and comfortable. OPPOSITE The tents and cabins weave their way through the desert. Dotted among the cactuses and palm trees and with the sea just a stone's throw away, they are an unobtrusive addition to the landscape.

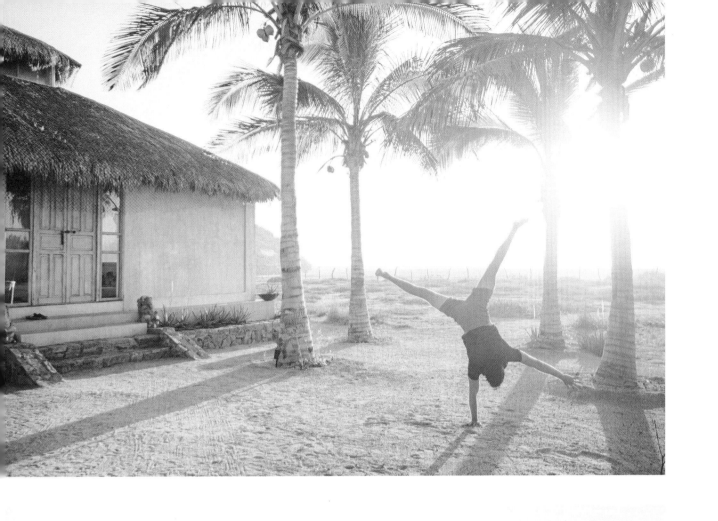
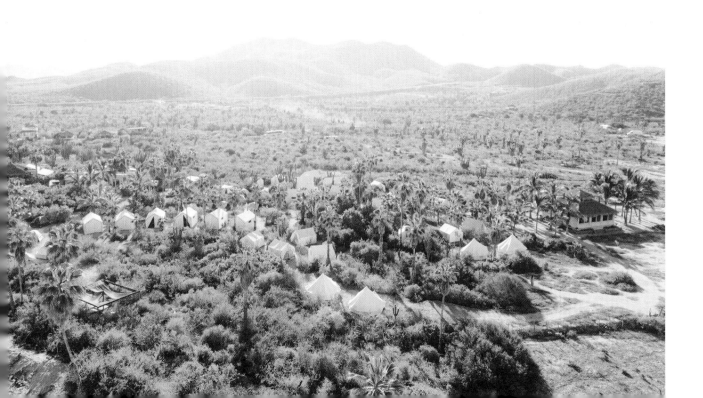

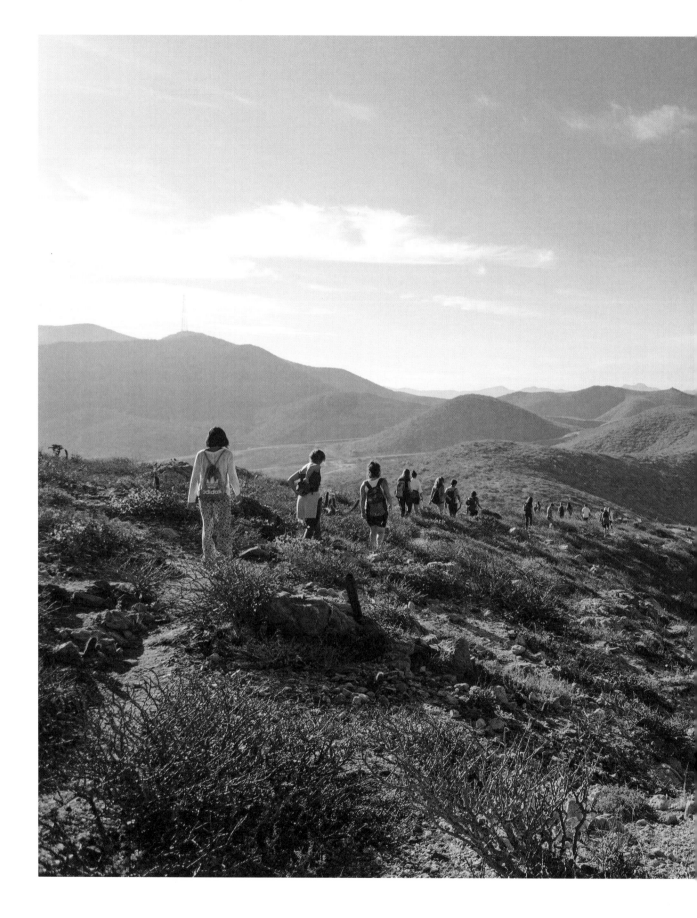

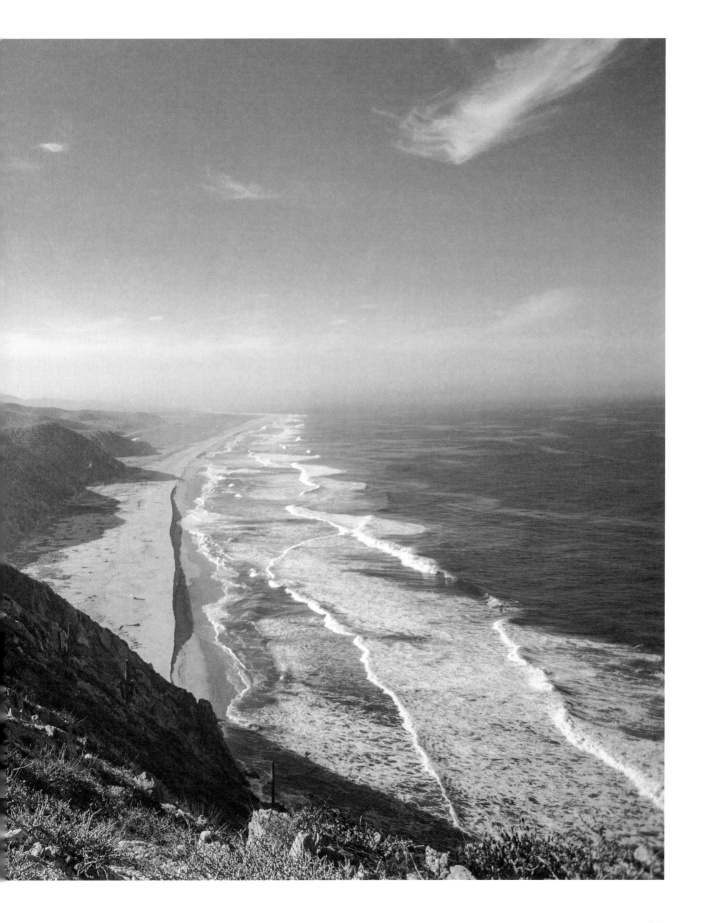

INDEX

RAGA SVARA
ragasvara.in
Rajkot, India
Photography courtesy of Raga Svara
pp. 58 – 63

SHE SHE RETREATS
sheshe-retreats.com
Deià, Mallorca, Spain
Photography: Ulrike Meutzner
ulrikemeutzner.com
pp. 10 – 17

SILVER ISLAND YOGA
silverislandyoga.com
Silver Island, Greece
Photography courtesy of
Silver Island Yoga
pp. 24 – 29

SON BLANC FARMHOUSE
sonblancmenorca.com
Menorca, Spain
Photography: Maria Missaglia
mariamissaglia.com
pp. 30, 32, 33 bottom
Karel Balas
karelbalas.com
pp. 33 top, 34, 35

STERREKOPJE FARM
sterrekopje.com
Franschhoek, Western Cape,
South Africa
Photography: Anne Timmer
annetimmer.com
pp. 6, 174, 179, 181
Gary van Wyk
garyvanwykphotography.com
p. 176 top
Sarah Frances Kelley
sarahfranceskelley.com
pp. 7 bottom, 176 bottom

Inge Prins
ingeprins.com
pp. 177, 178
Elsa Young
elsayoung.photography
p. 180
Emma Jude Jackson
emmajudejackson.com
pp. 182, 183

SUENYO ECO RETREAT
suenyo-bali.com
Tabanan, Bali, Indonesia
Photography courtesy of
Suenyo Eco Retreat
pp. 86 – 91

THE DWARIKA'S RESORT
dwarikas-dhulikhel.com
Dhulikhel, Nepal
Photography courtesy of
Dwarika's Resort
pp. 78, 81
Northabroad/Alexander Kinnunen
northabroad.com
pp. 80, 82 – 85

THE NEWT IN SOMERSET
thenewtinsomerset.com
Bruton, U.K.
Photography courtesy of
The Newt in Somerset
pp. 132 – 141

TIERRA PATAGONIA
tierrapatagonia.com
Torres del Paine, Chile
Photography courtesy of
Tierra Patagonia
pp. 160 – 165

VALE DE MOSES
valedemoses.com
Amieira, Portugal
Photography courtesy of
Vale de Moses
pp. 70 – 77

VILLA SUMAYA
villasumaya.com
Santa Cruz la Laguna, Guatemala
Photography courtesy of
Villa Sumaya
pp. 230 – 239

WYLDER IBIZA
wylder.net
San Miguel, Ibiza, Spain
Photography: Sofia Gomez Fonzo
sofiagomezfonzo.com
pp. 240 – 245
Marc Torres
theotherfaceibiza.com
pp. 246 – 247

YANDARA YOGA INSTITUTE
yandararetreats.com
Todos Santos, Mexico
Photography courtesy of
Yandara Yoga Institute
pp. 248 – 253

ZIEDLEJAS
ziedlejas.lv
Sigulda, Latvia
Photography: Alvis Rozenbergs
@alchsh
pp. 150 – 152, 154 – 159
Courtesy of Ziedlejas
p. 153

Mindful Places to Stay

Sublime Destinations for Yoga and Meditation

This book was conceived, edited, and designed by *gestalten*.

Edited by *Robert Klanten* and *Masha Erman*

Editorial support by *Effie Efthymiadi* and *Katharina Hegemann*

Introduction, project texts, and captions by *Anna Southgate*

Editorial Management: *Anna Diekmann* and *Arndt Jasper*
Photo Editor: *Zoe Paterniani*

Design, layout, and cover by *Joana Sobral*
Layout assistence by *Stefan Morgner*
Typefaces: Catull by *Gustav Jaeger* and Minion by *Robert Slimbach*

Cover image: courtesy of Silver Island Yoga
Backcover image: she she Retreats, photography by Ulrike Meutzner

Printed by Finidr, s.r.o, Český Těšín, Czech Republic
Made in Europe

Published by gestalten, Berlin 2024
ISBN 978-3-96704-146-0

© Die Gestalten Verlag GmbH & Co. KG, Berlin 2024

For more information, and to order books, please visit www.gestalten.com

Bibliographic information published by the Deutsche Nationalbibliothek.
The Deutsche Nationalbibliothek lists this publication in the Deutsche Nationalbibliografie;
detailed bibliographic data is available online at www.dnb.de

None of the content in this book was published in exchange for payment by commercial
parties or designers; the inclusion of all work is based solely on its artistic merit.

This book was printed on paper certified according to the standards of the FSC®.

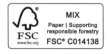

MIX
Paper | Supporting
responsible forestry
FSC® C014138